SUBTLE MEDICINE

Everything is a Play of Consciousness When Consciousness Becomes the Basis of Structure Three Intelligences and Three Tendencies Improving the Quality of Health Care from Within Becoming Aware of Mind-Body-Spirit Medicine Intuitive Medicine **Quantum View of Medicine and its Implications** Halting Dehumanization in Medicine Connecting with Spiritual Intelligence in Medicine **Consciousness as the basis of Disease and Disaster** Everything is a Play of Consciousness Becoming Aware of Mind-Body-Spirit Medicine **Quantum View of Medicine and its Implications** Connecting with Spiritual Intelligence in Medicine **Consciousness as the basis of Disease and Disaster** Everything is a Play of Consciousness When Consciousness Becomes the Basis of Structure Three Intelligences and Three Tendencies Improving the Quality of Health Care from Within Becoming Aware of Mind-Body-Spirit Medicine Intuitive Medicine **Quantum View of Medicine and its Implications** Halting Dehumanization in Medicine Clarity as against certainty in medicine Connecting with Spiritual Intelligence in Medicine **Consciousness as the basis of Disease and Disaster** Everything is a Play of Consciousness When Consciousness Becomes the Basis of Structure Three Intelligences and Three Tendencies Improving the Quality of Health Care from Within Becoming Aware of Mind-Body-Spirit Medicine Intuitive Medicine **Quantum View of Medicine and its Implications** Halting Dehumanization in Medicine Common platform for all systems of medicine Clarity as against Certainty in medicine The need for psycho-spiritual history in clinical medicine Outline for Empathy-Based Medical education When 'Ignorance is Bliss' in Medicine Science that swears by objectivity is half-blind The 'Inside-Out' Approach to Therapeutic Care

Dr. VIJAYARAGHAVAN PADMANABHAN MD

*This book is dedicated to
my parents Rajalakshmi and
Padmanabhan and to my
Divine Master
Sri Sathya Sai Baba*

Contents

#1 Health Care Needs a Fundamentally New Approach [7]
#2 The Unlimited Potential of Mind-Body-Spirit Medicine [18]
#3 Everything is a Play of Consciousness [20]
#4 Our Built-in Biofeedback [22]
#5 Understanding Meditation [24]
#6 Bliss Feedback Therapy [26]
#7 When Consciousness Becomes the Basis of Structure [28]
#8 Three Intelligences and Three Tendencies [30]
#9 Improving the Quality of Health Care from Within [34]
#10 Becoming Aware of Mind-Body-Spirit Medicine [40]
#11 Empathy, Research and the Medical Teacher [44]
#12 Fixing the Basic flaw in Medical Education and Health Care [49]
#13 Intuitive Medicine [52]
#14 Quantum View of Medicine and its Implications [56]
#15 The Need for Empathy-Based Medical Education [60]
#16 Halting Dehumanization in Medicine [64]
#17 Connecting with Spiritual Intelligence in Medicine [73]
#18 Consciousness as the basis of disease and disaster [80]
#19 A common platform for all systems of medicine [87]
#20 Clarity as against Certainty in Medicine [94]
#21 The need for psycho-spiritual history in clinical medicine [100]
#22 Outline for Empathy-Based Medical Education [104]
#23: When 'Ignorance is Bliss' in Medicine [110]
#24: Science that swears by objectivity is half-blind [114]
#25: The 'Inside-Out' Approach to Therapeutic Care [118]
BIBILIOGRAPHY [123]
ABOUT THE AUTHOR [125]
AFTERWORD [126]
BOOKS BY THIS AUTHOR [127]

FOREWORD

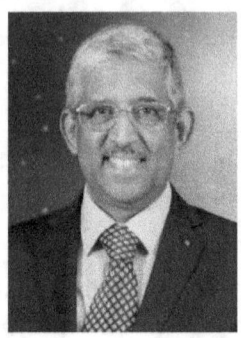

It gives me great pleasure to write this Foreword for my good friend and colleague Dr. Vijayaraghavan Padmanabhan. Dr. Vijayaraghavan, in a series of articles written by him, which he has collated in the form of a book, deals with a very difficult subject - the mind, body, spirit and medicine as he calls it. Today, healthcare has become a commodity and a few physicians think of a holistic approach to healthcare. Healthcare has also become fragmented because of the development of 'specialties' where one specialist thinks only of the heart, the other only of the brain and the other only of the disease in which they are specialized in. This often results not only in dissatisfaction from the patient's point of view because the individual is not treated as a whole, but as a sum of his or her parts. This often leads to wrong diagnosis as each specialist tends to think of only his or her specialty.

At a higher level, Dr. Vijayaraghavan dwells deeper into the mind and how it influences health as well as diseases. He makes a fervent plea for a holistic approach to health bringing in all the components as defined by the World

Health Organization (WHO) which defines Health as a state of complete physical, mental and social wellbeing and not merely the absence of disease or infirmity. Later, the WHO and other bodies also added the spiritual dimension to health. Our physical body is strongly influenced by the subconscious mind and both our physical as well as mental health is influenced by our deep thoughts which are in the sub-cortical region. The power of this subcortical brain is only beginning to be understood by physicians and scientists. However, our ancient masters and spiritual leaders knew the power of the mind and through intense yoga and meditation practices were able to perform cures on seemingly incurable diseases.

A complete understanding of all the dimensions of health including the spiritual dimension will not only result in a complete and wholesome treatment but also contribute to improved quality of life. It also leads to a sense of wellbeing which can only be experienced as it is very difficult to describe. In this modern era of mass commercialization and separatist tendencies in healthcare, Dr. Vijayaraghavan's book obviously inspired by his spiritual Guru and Master, Bhagawan Sri Sathya Sai Baba, is a much-needed book reflecting high philosophical ideals combined with practical healthcare. Being a physician himself, he is able to understand both sides of the coin. I would strongly recommend not only physicians, but everyone, to read this book as it is truly an eye opener. I wish Dr. Vijayaraghavan all the very best for the publication of this book and also look forward to many more such contributions from him.

Om Jai Sai Ram!

Dr. V. MOHAN, M.D., FRCP (London, Edinburgh, Glasgow, Ireland), Ph.D., D.Sc., D.Sc (Hon. Causa), FNASc, FASc, FNA, FACE, FTWAS, MACP, FRSE (Edinburgh)
Chairman & Chief Diabetologist, Dr. Mohan's Diabetes Specialties Centre &
President, Madras Diabetes Research Foundation, Chennai.
Member, Board of Trustees, Sri Sathya Sai Central Trust
[Dated: 26 March 2018]

#1: Health Care Needs a Fundamentally New Approach

Introduction: While modern medicine has made great strides, in terms of health care of the population, the diagnosis and treatment of diseases has become more complex and expensive while the disease burden remains high.

There is a lesson to be learnt from the many alternative systems of medicine, which consider mind-body-spirit as an integrated whole [1]. Because of their simplicity and demonstrated efficacy, these wholistic systems have become increasingly popular throughout the world. There is a general perception among academic circles that modern medicine complimented with alternative systems of medicine has therapeutic benefits. However, the reason why the wholistic systems work has not been enquired into.

The focus of this article is to show that there is enough scientific evidence for the presence of a spiritual dimension to the human structure and function, which accounts for the apparent success of 'mind-body-spirit' systems of medicine. The spiritual dimension when understood and harnessed has far reaching implications on how modern medicine is taught and, on the way, diseases are managed.

What is Health? The World Health Organization has defined health as a state of complete physical, mental and social wellbeing, and not merely the absence of disease or infirmity. Some people do enjoy such a state of complete wellbeing. Their life is in harmony with themselves as well as the world around them. They feel contentment and enjoy peace; they understand problems pertaining to themselves as well as the world around them and are inclined to solve them. This is the state of spiritual wellbeing, which can be felt and enjoyed but is difficult to be expressed in words. The state of complete physical, mental and social wellbeing referred to by the WHO, in reality implies an all-encompassing spiritual dimension perceivable by the individual.

Spiritual Dimension: Modern medicine is based on objective evidence. The physician makes use of knowledge based on the truth of science. The feeling of spiritual wellbeing is subjective truth, which is equally true from the physician's point of view. The epistemology or the grounds of knowledge may be different, yet it makes no difference from the point of view of application of that knowledge. While modern medicine offers solutions to problems affecting the tangible dimensions, due to epistemological reasons it is unable to consider health in its totality, which includes the spiritual dimension. It is left to the individual physician to grasp this subjective truth and suggest remedies to problems viewed best from this perspective. The emergence of stress-related diseases as a major problem in recent times has focused attention on the spiritual dimension [2].

The Basis for Spiritual Wellbeing: If spiritual dimension of health is a fact, then there should be a basis for it, just as body has matter as its basis and the mind has thought as its basis. The basis for spiritual dimension is a subtle faculty within us called Spiritual Intelligence. While cognitive intelligence (IQ) is about 'thinking' and emotional intelligence (EQ) is about 'feeling', spiritual intelligence (SQ) is about 'being' [3]. Acquiring an integrated view of oneself and the environment is necessary for the individual's feeling of contentment or the bliss of 'being'. This bliss of 'being' may be termed as spiritual bliss to distinguish it from sensory bliss or bliss related to the senses.

Spiritual intelligence comes into play whenever the individual dwells on his 'self' or 'the individual's perceived reality', a process that happens on and off and underlies our consciousness. The 'inner self' (also called 'pure consciousness' or 'Self') is reached and experienced as pure bliss in deep sleep. While the 'self' perceives duality, and is subject to a variety of feelings, the 'inner self' perceives unity and experiences pure bliss. Once this core reality of blissful 'being' is reached, all information in a person's life is reconciled around it. A person waking up after a good deep sleep feels refreshed and blissful. This feeling of pure bliss fades once the individual starts perceiving the world of duality. Shortfall in the process of reconciliation around the core of pure bliss, results in stress or absence of spiritual wellbeing.

Maintaining Spiritual Wellbeing: Thus, we understand that the state of spiritual wellbeing and the total health encompassed by it ultimately rests on our spiritual intelligence, though most of us are not aware of this faculty. A person in normal health subconsciously maintains his spiritual wellbeing through his built-in spiritual intelligence. He is able to enjoy the bliss of his 'self', which is refreshed and sustained by the pure bliss of his 'inner self'. However spiritual intelligence can also be voluntarily cultivated to heal stress related disorders [4]. Meditation is basically a method of cultivating spiritual intelligence. It is a method of consciously transcending one's 'self' to reach the 'inner self'. Meditation enables the individual to perceive in reality the pure bliss of the 'inner self'. A fleeting perception of this bliss occurs in the twilight zone between a good sleep and the fully awake state. Keeping the mind focused on this subtle perception of pure bliss is a simple method of meditation that can be practiced by all. Constant contemplation of the pure bliss of 'inner self' helps to restore spiritual wellbeing and heal stress.

While we understand the value of meditation for healing stress in a given patient, we also gain insight on how physician's themselves can enjoy lasting spiritual wellbeing and thus stand to gain personally and professionally by practicing the technique of meditation in their daily lives.

The Pathophysiology of Diseases: While the disruption of spiritual bliss and its healing through the process of meditation can be easily appreciated in stress-related disorders, the new science of psychoneuroimmunology indicates that spiritual wellbeing needs to be taken into consideration while understanding the pathogenesis of nearly every disease [5][6][7], including the so-called physical diseases. Studies indicate that the psycho-neuro-immuno axis is at work in many disease states and this may determine the outcome of disease processes [8][9]. Since the state of the mind largely depends on the state of spiritual wellbeing, it is evident that all diseases need to be considered not merely from the body or mind-body perspective but from a wholistic mind-body-spirit perspective.

The Art of Healing: It is well known that good practice of medicine is both a science as well as an art. The 'art of healing' [10] largely depends on the quality of empathy [11] present in a physician. A compassionate physician presumably acts a catalyst for healing through the patient's own built-in mechanisms. The role of the physician in providing the humane touch is crucial, which cannot be replaced by any technology. Being a good listener, speaking a few kind words and spending a few more minutes with a sincere body language may be all that is needed to have a healing effect on the 'self' of the patient. Modern medicine becomes 'modern mind-body-spirit medicine' when the physician incorporates the 'art of healing' in his professional practice.

From being considered merely as a desirable virtue, it is time for the 'art of healing' to be considered as a basic component in any attempt to restore normal health from a diseased state [12]. Ignoring this fact and viewing disease merely from a body or a mind-body perspective would amount to intervening into a problem that may be causally downstream while a possible cause upstream is left unattended. The current bio-medical approach, which considers body and the mind as the basis of health is truth but not the whole truth.

Medicine - the present and the future: The world of medicine today is based on scientific lines and the quality of empathy is considered desirable among health care providers rather than as a basic necessity. The bio-medical approach to health and disease has made the delivery of health care predominantly lab-oriented and mechanical. Valuable resources are spent for understanding the physical aspects of disease, while the bigger picture that includes the spiritual dimension is neglected. Increasing technological sophistication is valued more than the therapeutic potential of physician's compassion. As a result, tertiary care gets preference over primary care. The society as well as the medical professionals themselves, finds physician-based primary care unattractive.

Inevitably, the consequence of this is felt in the way medicine is taught to students. An impersonal 'matter of fact' approach is appropriate to teach the physical, mental and social aspects of diseases. In the absence of an academic framework to teach the spiritual aspect, students are not briefed about it and frequently fail to gain spiritual insight. Setting a personal example by practicing the 'art of healing' while treating patients is an effective way of teaching the spiritual aspect. However, in the academic setting there is need for this effort to be supplemented by a curriculum that is built around the core of the individual's spiritual wellbeing. The importance of cultivating and maintaining spiritual wellbeing by the physician himself so that he can practice the 'art of healing' needs to be emphasized.

Conclusion: The basis of health and the pathogenesis of diseases have subtle spiritual underpinnings necessitating an integrated mind-body-spirit model of health and disease. The importance of spiritual wellbeing of the patient, its influence on the mind and consequently on the healing process of the body have been highlighted by recent advances in psychoneuroimmunology.

Disease management becomes more effective if the patient's own immune mechanisms are harnessed through the age-old 'art of healing'. Medical education being a key input in disease management needs to be suitably modified to emphasize the central role of spiritual wellbeing and the value of the practice of meditation by the physicians themselves.

Modern medicine is at cross-roads. With further scientific developments modern medicine would continue to benefit from newer technologies. At the same time, what is immediately required to improve the effectiveness of modern medicine and decrease health care costs would be to formally integrate the 'art of healing' with the science of medicine. Incorporating the philosophy of mind-body-spirit medicine within the medical curriculum and health care structures would, in addition, place the job of the primary care physician at a higher level. Health care thus needs a fundamentally new approach to address the twin problems of escalation of costs and increasing neglect of primary care.

References:

1. Seaward BL. Alternative medicine complements standard. Various forms focus on holistic concepts. Health Prog.1994 Sep; 75(7): 52-7.

http://www.ncbi.nlm.nih.gov/entrez/query.f

cgi?cmd=Retrieve&db=pubmed&do
pt=Abstract&list_uids=10136081&q
uery_hl=13

2. Seaward BL. Stress and human spirituality 2000: at the cross roads of physics and metaphysics. Appl Psychophysiol Biofeedback. 2000 Dec; 25(4): 241- 6.
http://www.ncbi.nlm.nih.gov/entrez/query.f
cgi?cmd=Retrieve&db=pubmed&do
pt=Abstract&list_uids=11218925

3. Brian McMullen. Spiritual Intelligence. Student BMJ 2003 March; 11:60-61
http://archive.student.bmj.com/search/pdf/
03/03/sbmj60.pdf

4. Suzanne Davidson. Cultivating spiritual intelligence to heal diseases of meaning: A conference report. Contemporary Nurse 2002 Apr; 12(2):103
http://www.contemporarynurse.com/archive
s/vol/12/issue/2/article/1812/cultivating-
spiritual-intelligence-to-heal

5. Mausch K. The Psyche, the Immunological system and the problems of Health and Disease. Psychiatr Pol. 1995 Jul-Aug;29(4):435-41.
http://www.ncbi.nlm.nih.gov/pubmed/7568
516?ordinalpos=2&itool=EntrezSystem2.
PEntrez.Pubmed.Pubmed_ResultsPanel.Pubm
ed_DefaultReportPanel.Pubmed_RVDocSum

6. Lutgendorf SK, Costanzo ES. Psychoneuroimmunology and health psychology: an integrative model. Brain Behav Immun. 2003 Aug; 17(4): 225-32.
http://www.ncbi.nlm.nih.gov/entrez/query.fcgi?cmd=Retrieve&db=pubmed&dopt=Abstract&list_uids=12831823

7. Kiecolt-Glaser JK, McGuire L, Robles TF, Glaser R. Emotions, morbidity and mortality: new perspectives from psychoneuroimmunology. Annu Rev Psychol. 2002; 53:83-107.
http://www.ncbi.nlm.nih.gov/entrez/query.fcgi?cmd=Retrieve&db=pubmed&dopt=Abstract&list_uids=11752480

8. Kiecolt-Glaser JK, Glaser R. Psychoneuroimmunology and cancer: fact or fiction? European Journal of Cancer. 1999 Oct; 35(11):1603-7.
http://www.ncbi.nlm.nih.gov/entrez/query.fcgi?cmd=Retrieve&db=pubmed&dopt=Abstract&list_uids=10673969

9. Robinson FP, Mathews HL, Witek-Janusek L. Stress reduction and HIV disease: a review of intervention studies using a psychoneuroimmunology framework. J Assoc Nurses AIDS Care. 2000 Mar-Apr; 11(2): 87-96.
http://www.ncbi.nlm.nih.gov/entrez/query.fcgi?cmd=Retrieve&db=pubmed&dopt=Abstract&list_uids=10752051

10. Bernard Lown: The Lost Art of Healing. BMJ 1997 (20 Sept.); 315:755
http://bmj.bmjjournals.com/cgi/content/full/315/7110/755

11. Heidenreich KS. Empathy in the physician-patient relation: tool or ethics? Tidsskr Nor Laegeforen 2001 May 10; 121(12): 1507-11.
http://www.ncbi.nlm.nih.gov/entrez/query.fcgi?cmd=Retrieve&db=pubmed&dopt=Abstract&list_uids=11449777

12. Recognizing the Mind/Body/Spirit Connection in Medical Care. Samuel E. Karff, DHL. Virtual Mentor. Oct 2009, Vol 11, No 10: 788-792
http://virtualmentor.ama-assn.org/2009/10/msoc1-0910.html

#2: The Unlimited Potential of Mind-Body-Spirit Medicine

There is increasing scientific evidence (especially in the developing field of psychoneuroimmunology) for a rational basis for the concept of Mind-Body-Spirit medicine. It is also termed as Era 3 medicine, Era 1 being Body and Era 2 being Mind-Body medicine.

However, Mind-Body-Spirit medicine is best viewed as a philosophy where the mind, the body and the spirit are viewed as an integrated whole. Mind-Body-Spirit integrity is actually an age-old concept being fundamental to Ayurveda and other similar systems that come under the category of Alternative medicine.

Those of us who have been educated in the modern scientific way, trained in Physics Chemistry and Biology, find it difficult to accept the intuitive way of understanding the concept of spirit. We find the logical way of understanding matters, sensible. We tend to discard anything that is not supported by logic. In fact, our intuitive mind has regressed.

Accepting the philosophy of Mind-Body-Spirit medicine requires a developed intuitive mind that is balanced by the logical mind. Intuitive mind is simply the ability to feel within oneself the nature of a problem or thing. Though every one of us has this in-born faculty and make use of it, we are trained by science to use our logical mind to understand matters.

The learning and teaching of conventional biomedical approach to health and disease consists of understanding the structure and function conveyed through words. Deeper understanding implies assimilating more information. It mainly depends upon the efficacy of the logical aspect of mind.

Understanding and applying the philosophy of mind-body-spirit medicine depends mainly on the intuitive aspect of mind. Assimilation of more and more information is not a priority. Instead, understanding the soul of the patient through the faculty of empathy is a primary requirement. In fact, assimilating more information beyond a limit may be deleterious to the physician's faculty of empathy.

The physician understands the patient as a person and then utilizes the information about the disease process to the extent needed and prescribes his treatment. Mind-body-spirit medicine allows the unknown to be tackled by the body's built-in mechanisms. Thus, the therapeutic potential of mind-body-spirit medicine is unlimited, while the purely biomedical approach confines itself to limits set by the logical mind.

#3: Everything is a Play of Consciousness

Take for instance a typical day in the life of an individual. When the person wakes up in the morning the world comes into existence as far as he (or she) is concerned. If he feels bliss within himself after a nice deep sleep, he tends to feel happiness in the world around him. He is unaffected by problems around him, but tries to solve them if possible. His entire day feels positive and productive.

On the other hand, if the same person wakes up after a poor sleep, he lacks bliss in his heart and his 'mood' is not so good. He tends to get affected by problems around him. He may even compound the existing problems rather than helping to solve them. He may wish that the day ends soon.

What matters here is how the person feels at the moment of his awakening. The state of his conscious mind when he starts perceiving the world, determines the quality of the rest of the day for him. That 'consciousness', whether it is blissful or lacks bliss, is the basis upon which his day is built. All other things are secondary.

Once this foundation - the principle of consciousness - is understood then we have a way to influence the state of our own consciousness and the quality of our day. All we have to do is to ensure that we have a nice sound sleep by avoiding things/thoughts that can disturb our feeling of happiness during the previous day.

Once we have a good sleep the next day dawns well and it is easier to maintain the feeling of happiness on subsequent days, provided we do not fall prey to negative emotions that can disturb us. One way of perpetuating happiness is to keep contemplating on the bliss that persists for some time after a good night's sleep during the course of the day.

When we understand that everything in a day's life is a play of consciousness then we ourselves can play with our consciousness. Control of consciousness leads to better control of mind. Better control of the mind means better control of what is done with the body and better health of the individual.

#4: Our Built-in Biofeedback

In the article titled - "Everything is a Play of Consciousness", the point was made that the state of our consciousness at the moment of our awakening from sleep, determines the quality of life for the rest of the day. If we feel blissful at the moment of awakening, then it is perpetuated for the rest of the day. If bliss is lacking then the whole day feels indifferent or even miserable.

This phenomenon is due to an in-built mechanism where the mind keeps coming back to the 'perceived reality' for that day, which is the state of our consciousness at the time of awakening. This forms the 'core consciousness' or the 'self' of that individual for that day, with all activities of the mind having this core as the basis.

The mind judges the events of the day with this core as the reference point. If the core is blissful then the mind also sees the world as basically blissful. When confronted by problems the feedback from the core anchors the mind to the 'blissful reality' and the mind overcomes problems by creating solutions.

This biofeedback from the 'core consciousness' maintains the quality of our consciousness, whether blissful or not. The mechanism of our built-in biofeedback explains why positive thinking works. See good, be good and do good may appear to be a moral advice to lead a happy blissful life, but it has a biological basis.

#5: Understanding Meditation

It was explained in the previous article that the concept of 'self' or the 'perceived reality' of an individual, is about the state of his consciousness at the time of awakening from sleep. This 'self' persists and influences the quality of that particular day through 'our built-in biofeedback'. The emphasis is on the presence or absence of the quality of bliss.

Blissfulness is the core quality that would determine the expression of other faculties of the mind. When a person is blissful, his mind is calm and his intellect and judgment is optimal. Blissfulness is the natural quality of the 'self' as is evident in children. Being blissful allows all other human faculties to blossom.

As grownups many of us would feel far removed from bliss. This is because we allow the mind and its senses to dwell upon so many things in our day-to-day lives. Thus the 'self' or the 'perceived reality', even if it is blissful soon after a good night's sleep, soon forgets this core reality of bliss.

The problem is to recover from this 'superimposed reality' that is lacking in bliss and reach back again to the 'self' that is blissful. Our mind should release itself from the problems of the day and start dwelling on the inner 'self' that is hidden from consciousness.

Many would be able to do this involuntarily by just relaxing and going to sleep. On reaching the deep sleep state, freed from thoughts and input from the senses the individual experiences pure bliss.

But in today's world more and more people find it difficult to get released from the thoughts of the day. To overcome this problem, several techniques of relaxation and meditation are available. The individual may choose the particular technique that appeals to him most.

A simplified understanding of meditation is - it is basically the process of consciously transcending the 'apparent self' to reach the 'inner self', which is blissful.

#6: Bliss Feedback Therapy

The previous articles dwelt on the terms – 'consciousness', 'apparent self', 'inner self' and the process of 'meditation'. The feeling of bliss, which is formless, is perceived and sustained by the individual through the 'built-in biofeedback'.

During the process of meditation, when the individual consciously tries to reach the bliss of the 'inner self', he uses a framework to perceive the formless bliss. A sensory perception, usually visual or auditory, that is associated with inner bliss is made use of by the mind. This 'associate' of bliss depends on the method of meditation.

A pitfall in meditation is to start believing this 'associate' of bliss as real, pushing the bliss itself to the background. Individuals may be practicing a particular method of meditation in a mechanical way forgetting the bliss. True meditation would always focus on the bliss, which is the essence.

Philosophically speaking, all religions help individuals to reach their blissful 'inner self'. They use auditory or visual frameworks to help the individual to perceive the bliss within oneself. If this primary purpose of religion is understood, then the apparent 'rituals' of religion become more meaningful.

Once established in bliss, the framework is no longer needed. However, since we are frequently distanced from bliss, we need to be re-established in bliss by constantly remembering the framework that is associated with bliss. With guidance and by practice, reaching and remaining in a state of bliss becomes easier.

Enjoying a state of bliss implies that the mind, body and the spirit are in an optimal state of health. The quality of sleep is good and this ensures a whole lot of health benefits. Any disease that might have set in heals faster when the individual practices meditation. Meditation may thus be called as 'bliss feedback therapy'.

#7: When Consciousness Becomes the Basis of Structure

We have seen how one can modify one's state of consciousness by the method of meditation. One's life can be positively influenced and the state of health improved. This implies that physical manifestations of disease are also positively modified by sustained maintenance of the state of consciousness at a blissful level. Thus, consciousness becomes the basis of structure of the body.

Therefore, the assumption that structure is the basis of consciousness is not always true. It can be the other way around. When it is understood that the state of consciousness can lead to changes in structure, it opens a new way of understanding the basis of disease and health.

Presently science is discovering the genetic basis of several disease processes. The gene mutations responsible for specific diseases help in tracing carrier states and in predicting the likelihood of an individual or his/her offspring to develop a particular disease.

Since the structure-consciousness link can work the other way around, one can postulate that changes in consciousness can produce modifications in the gene structure. When a person develops a particular behavior due to social circumstances, with no family history of similar behavior, it is possible that gene modifications take place. For example, the habit of smoking has a genetic basis [1]. However, when a person develops the habit of smoking when there is no family history of smoking, it is possible that modifications in gene structure take place. The liking for smoking may then be transmitted to his off-spring genetically.

References:

1. Genetic basis of tobacco smoking: strong association of a specific major histocompatibility complex haplotype on chromosome 6 with smoking behavior. Füst G Arason GJ Kramer J et. al. Int Immunol. 2004 Oct;16(10):1507-14. Epub 2004 Aug 31.
https://www.ncbi.nlm.nih.gov/pubmed/1533 9882

#8: Three Intelligences and Three Tendencies

The concepts of 'perceived reality' and 'inner reality' of an individual denoting the 'self' and 'inner self' have been dealt with in the earlier articles. The individual spends the day in the 'perceived reality', which is practically speaking, the state of consciousness at the time of awakening from sleep. During the phase of deep sleep, the mind reaches the indefinable 'inner reality' or 'pure consciousness', which can be understood as the bliss of deep sleep. Upon waking up the individual enjoys the left-over of this bliss, which is carried with the 'consciousness' of the day and determines its quality.

Broadly speaking, the individual's consciousness is capable of three types of 'knowing' or cognition or intelligence, namely, that perceived by the logical mind, that perceived by feeling and that perceived by the core of one's 'being'. Popularly they have come to be known as IQ, EQ and SQ. General Intelligence or IQ was the first to be recognized, which could be evaluated through psychometric tests. Later Emotional Intelligence or EQ was found to be even more important for the individual's success in his daily life or profession. Spiritual Intelligence or SQ has recently been recognized as the most basic of all the three, which determines success in the individual's life as a whole.

Through Spiritual Intelligence (synonymous with 'conscience at work'), all 'knowing' by the individual is reconciled around the core of one's 'self' (the 'inner self' or simply 'being'). When the reconciliation is complete, the mind easily reaches and enjoys the bliss of deep sleep. In the deep sleep state, there is only this bliss of 'being' with the various intelligences remaining un-manifest. When the 'being' becomes 'becoming', the consciousness of the waking state carries with it this bliss. Thus 'being' still lies within 'becoming', when the intelligences are at work.

There is the 'source' or 'being' or the 'inner self'. Spiritual Intelligence works closest to the 'source' and requires deep inner awareness to be appreciated. Emotional Intelligence comes further downstream, requires lesser inner awareness and is more easily appreciated. General Intelligence comes last and is widely appreciated in daily life. When the individual or the 'self' is blissful, the working of the intelligences is optimal and imperceptible. When the 'self' is less than blissful, the first to be affected is Spiritual Intelligence; next comes Emotional Intelligence. General Intelligence is preserved unless the individual is severely disturbed.

When the individual is aware of only his General Intelligence, he would consider acquiring more knowledge in his area of work to be the key for success in life. If he becomes aware of his Emotional

Intelligence, he would consider 'feeling' to be more important than 'thinking'. When the individual is aware of his Spiritual Intelligence there is realization that the quality of everything downstream depends on the bliss of 'being'. He finds that by meditating on the bliss of 'being' control is maintained on everything downstream, which in turn has a subtle effect on life as a whole. He enjoys blissfulness in his life and the various intelligences work to serve his purpose.

The above narrated process of enjoying blissfulness is compounded by three tendencies the individual has to reckon with. The 'perceived reality' or 'self' of the individual is determined by the interplay of these three tendencies, in-born within each individual in differing proportions and accounting for the diversity in the nature of individuals. Awareness of these tendencies is needed for the individual to proceed upstream and meditate on the 'source' or the bliss of 'being' instead of getting lost in the tantalizing manifestations of the external world. The three tendencies (or qualities) are the serene, the active and the passive.

Of these three, the serene tendency if dominant helps the individual to acquire closeness with the bliss of 'being'. The active tendency leads the individual towards exploration and action entangling him with the phenomena of the objective world. The passive tendency if dominant leads the individual towards sensory pleasure and sloth. The serene tendency uniquely heals the disturbances arising out of the other two tendencies and if lacking leads to stress and its consequences. A healthy balance between these three tendencies helps the individual to lead a healthy and productive life.

The serene tendency is the foundation upon which the expansion of the active tendency and the enjoyment of the passive tendency rest. The cause of much of the ill-health found in individuals and society lies in loss of balance between these three tendencies. While the active and passive tendencies are glorified in every-day life, the serene tendency is relegated to the realm of spirituality and not considered essential. Understanding the working of these three tendencies and giving due importance to the foundation or the serene tendency is essential for restoration of health.

#9: Improving the Quality of Health Care from Within

The starting as well as the central point of any healing is the faith that the patient has for the doctor. Implied in this is the patient's belief that the best treatment under the circumstances is being given to heal the disease he (or she) is suffering from. When the patient is content about this, he is prepared to wait for the disease to improve and to face whatever problems that may be encountered. The reassuring words from the physician strengthens his faith.

This faith that the patient has, can also involve faith in the institution or hospital where he is undergoing treatment. He believes that the place where he has come seeking relief would finally turn out to be good for him. Faith also matters in the case of a child or an invalid who believes that his parent or guardian is taking care of him. Faith is a deep-seated feeling that leads to contentment and soothes the questioning mind.

Faith is essential for healing to take place regardless of the kind of treatment that is actually given. Without faith the mind is active and restless. This has repercussions on the immune system. The new field of psychoneuroimmunology [1-5] has validated the reality of mind-body-spirit medicine [6-9]. Where there is faith, the feeling is positive and this helps the body's built-in mechanisms of healing.

Therefore, a basic requirement for a successful health outcome would be to ensure that the care given at the healthcare setting strengthens the faith of the patient. The physician should live up to the faith reposed in him by arriving at the cause of the disease process just as the archer aims at the 'bull's eye'. He needs to use his medical knowledge and clinical acumen to zero-in on the cause as soon as possible and start the appropriate treatment. The rest of the healing should be left to the body's built-in mechanisms; or in lay-man's term - to 'nature'. It is unnecessary as well as virtually impossible to understand and 'utilize' every mechanism underlying 'nature'.

The central role of faith has implications on how medicine is taught to students. The young medico needs to learn the bio-medical aspects by acquiring a sound knowledge of the basic sciences. Even as he learns the basics of clinical examination, he needs to learn the art of dealing with the patient and his concerns. He needs to understand the central role of faith in healing and that his own medical knowledge and skill only help to supplement the body's built-in mechanisms of healing.

Post-graduate learning in medicine should concentrate on the student's ability to manage various disease conditions and lead to perfection of clinical acumen. Acquiring more and more theoretical knowledge of diseases without actual case management is of little use and would only serve to distract the budding physician from developing the habit of targeting the 'bull's eye'. Sir William Osler's well-known emphasis on learning medicine by the bedside acquires added importance in the context of the new-found validity of mind-body-spirit medicine.

Presently modern medicine does not recognize the role of faith and the reality of mind-body-spirit medicine. Relying purely on the bio-medical aspects has led to a mechanical approach to diseases with loss of human touch. In addition, there is uncertainty in the face of rapid medical advances, on how much of medicine is to be learnt and how best to evaluate the newly qualifying doctors.

The quality of health care would eventually depend on how well the roles of the health care professional, health care facilities, medical advances and medical education are synchronized to supplement and support the central nature of faith and the hidden reality of mind-body-spirit medicine. Otherwise, the different aspects of health care would remain as disparate entities, one contradicting the other. For example, doctors may know the value of spending time with the patient and making a good clinical diagnosis, but may not be in a position to follow it in practice because of the necessity to make use of inappropriately built-up diagnostic facilities.

In these times of escalating health care costs and

sorry state of national health services, quality health care for all is still attainable if the basics are got right.

References:

1. Mausch K. The Psyche, the Immunological system and the problems of Health and Disease. Psychiatr Pol. 1995 Jul-Aug;29(4):435-41.
http://www.ncbi.nlm.nih.gov/pubmed/7568516?ordinalpos=2&itool=EntrezSystem2.PEntrez.Pubmed.Pubmed_ResultsPanel.Pubmed_DefaultReportPanel.Pubmed_RVDocSum

2. Lutgendorf SK, Costanzo ES. Psychoneuroimmunology and health psychology: an integrative model. Brain Behav Immun. 2003 Aug; 17(4): 225-32.
http://www.ncbi.nlm.nih.gov/entrez/query.fcgi?cmd=Retrieve&db=pubmed&dopt=Abstract&list_uids=12831823

3. Kiecolt-Glaser JK, McGuire L, Robles TF, Glaser R. Emotions, morbidity and mortality: new perspectives from psychoneuroimmunology. Annu Rev Psychol. 2002; 53:83-107.
http://www.ncbi.nlm.nih.gov/entrez/query.fcgi?cmd=Retrieve&db=pubmed&dopt=Abstract&list_uids=11752480

4. Kiecolt-Glaser JK, Glaser R. Psychoneuroimmunology and cancer: fact or

fiction? European Journal of Cancer. 1999 Oct; 35(11):1603-7.
http://www.ncbi.nlm.nih.gov/entrez/query.fcgi?cmd=Retrieve&db=pubmed&dopt=Abstract&list_uids=10673969

5. Robinson FP, Mathews HL, Witek-Janusek L. Stress reduction and HIV disease: a review of intervention studies using a psychoneuroimmunology framework. J Assoc Nurses AIDS Care. 2000 Mar-Apr; 11(2): 87-96
http://www.ncbi.nlm.nih.gov/entrez/query.fcgi?cmd=Retrieve&db=pubmed&dopt=Abstract&list_uids=10752051

6. Seaward BL. Alternative medicine complements standard. Various forms focus on holistic concepts. Health Prog. 1994 Sep; 75 (7) : 52-7.
http://www.ncbi.nlm.nih.gov/entrez/query.fcgi?cmd=Retrieve&db=pubmed&dopt=Abstract&list_uids=10136081&query_hl=13

7. Seaward BL. Stress and human spirituality 2000: at the cross roads of physics and metaphysics. Appl Psychophysiol Biofeedback. 2000 Dec; 25(4): 241-6.
http://www.ncbi.nlm.nih.gov/entrez/query.fcgi?cmd=Retrieve&db=pubmed&dopt=Abstract&list_uids=11218925

8. Brian McMullen. Spiritual Intelligence. Student

BMJ 2003 March; 11:60-61
http://archive.student.bmj.com/search/pdf/
03/03/sbmj60.pdf

9. Recognizing the Mind/Body/Spirit Connection in Medical Care. Samuel E. Karff, DHL. Virtual Mentor. Oct 2009, Vol 11, No 10: 788-792
http://virtualmentor.ama-assn.org/2009/10/msoc1-0910.html

#10: Becoming Aware of Mind-Body-Spirit Medicine

There are apparently two aspects of mind-body-spirit medicine that need to be understood. First is the hidden reality of mind-body-spirit medicine working through the body's built-in mechanisms of healing as brought out in the article 'Improving the quality of health care from within' [1]. Briefly, faith is essential for healing to take place regardless of the kind of treatment that is actually given. Without faith the mind is active and restless. This has repercussions on the immune system. Where there is faith, the feeling is positive and this helps the body's built-in mechanisms of healing.

The second aspect of mind-body-spirit medicine is the power of prayer or prayerful attitude to effect healing, in a non-local manner. This has been proved in numerous scientific studies and first brought to light with clarity by Dr. Larry Dossey, M.D. [2]. He calls this aspect of 'mind-body-spirit' medicine as the Era 3 medicine, Era 1 being 'body medicine' and Era 2 being 'mind-body medicine'. Dr. Larry points out that the key aspect of prayerfulness is empathy, caring, compassion or love. The experiments do not work well if there is no empathy, caring, compassion or love for the subject they are trying to influence.

The key to the patient developing faith is the empathy of the physician for the patient. The body's built-in mechanisms respond to the empathy or compassion of the physician. And Dr. Larry points out that empathy or compassion works in a non-local manner even if the patient is half way across the globe. Thus, empathy is central to mind-body-spirit medicine and it works in both the ways mentioned above. Those who naturally have the feeling of empathy towards patients and people in general, are at an advantage with regard to practicing mind-body-spirit medicine.

Interestingly the concepts of body, mind-body and mind-body-spirit medicine reinforces our understanding of ourselves. The development from Era 1 to Era 2 medicine emphasizes that we are not the body alone; we are mind-body entities. Era 3 medicine indicates that we are not confined to our mind-body. We are mind-body-spirit entities not bounded by distance. Our influence is trans-personal, non-local as proven by the studies on the effect of prayer.

As is the belief, so is the practice. If the physician believed that his own basis was merely the body, he would practice mostly Era 1 - plain mechanical medicine. If the physician believed that he was a mind-body entity, he would be practicing aspects of Era 2 medicine by giving importance to positive thinking. If the physician believed that he was a mind-body-spirit entity, he would include Era 3 medicine in his practice by giving importance to the attitude of 'prayerfulness' by whomsoever is concerned with the patient.

Thus, the three eras of medicine, though defined as starting from 1860, 1940 and 1990 (by Dr. Larry Dossey), must have been existing for a long time depending on what the physician (and the patient) believed himself to be -- whether he is predominantly physical, mental or a spiritual entity. In the present day, most physicians probably practice all three eras of medicine to varying extent since each complements the other. The type of patient (his predominant belief) and the circumstances of treatment may influence the physician to move between different eras in a given case.

The practice of 'mind-body-spirit medicine' or 'mind-body medicine' is not something that is contradictory to 'body medicine'. Awareness of the three eras by the physician leads to meaningful use of available approaches and more comprehensive patient care. While it makes assimilation of positive aspects of alternate medicine quite natural, the pure 'body medicine' approach to medical practice appears artificial and unnecessarily complicated. All three eras of medicine will continue to coexist as long as there are physicians (and patients) with differing awareness of themselves.

References:

1. Improving the Quality of Health Care from Within
http://www.futurehealth.org/populum/page.php?f=Improving-the-Quality-of-H-by-Vijayaraghavan-Pad-110501-893.html

2. A Conversation about the Future of Medicine
http://www.dosseydossey.com/larry/QnA.html

#11: Empathy, Research and the Medical Teacher

In recent times, it is recognized that the quality of empathy is crucial for the successful delivery of health care [1]. Empathy is a natural quality present in every medical student that needs to be fostered along with academics. It is known that students in the final year no longer feel as empathetic as they were when they joined the first year of medical course [2,3]. The cause for the decline in empathy lies in the structure of modern medicine that is based on the laws of physical sciences requiring the use of predominantly logical thinking and action. Since subjectivity has to be excluded to learn objectively there is little room for development of subjective feeling leading to a neglect of intuition and empathy. Because of the tendency for decline of empathy during the course of medical education, several methods have been suggested to improve empathy among students and physicians [4].

Adding to the factors contributing to decline of empathy is the lack of understanding of the three psychological aspects of being a doctor: (1) Doctor treating the patient (Medical Practitioner), (2) Doctor updating himself to treat better (Continuing Medical Education) and (3) Doctor analyzing data and understanding new aspects of diseases and their treatment (Research).

The first aspect of treating the patient is the basic

urge that drives the student to take up the career of medical profession. This interest in treating patients is what the society first expects from the medical profession. The purpose of medical education is to train doctors who can treat patients having different diseases with *competence and compassion*. The first task of the regulatory authorities should expectedly be to ensure that the medical colleges are equipped with appropriately qualified manpower (as well as infrastructure) to carry out this task.

The second aspect of being a doctor is the urge to keep abreast with new developments in the medical field so that he/she is able to improve the care given to the patients. This is a desirable trait and every doctor naturally has this to a greater or lesser extent. However, for a qualified doctor who is already equipped with compassion and basic competence, the need to update oneself with medical knowledge is arguably best left to his/her own judgment.

The third aspect is the urge to learn from the information available while treating patients to understand unknown aspects of diseases and devise new treatment. Many doctors do this either by observation of patients over years or by methodically collecting data in designed studies, analyzing them and publishing their findings in journals.

The first aspect of being a competent and

compassionate doctor does not depend on the second aspect of being updated with latest knowledge and even less on the third aspect of having interest in research and publication. Individual doctors who may be good in research may be found lacking in the ability to adequately care for the patient and *vice versa*, since different skills are required for these two functions.

When the regulatory bodies for medical education and practice do not understand the above three psychological aspects of being a doctor, it spells trouble. Though familiarity with research is needed, making publication of research papers compulsory for deciding the standing of a medical teacher seeks to whitewash all medical teachers into one category of having the capacity to do research whether or not they have the core capability of providing adequate patient-care. In reality there is heterogeneity of medical teachers; some are good in patient care, some in doing research. Medical students learn different sets of skills from different teachers.

Given the central importance of empathy in patient care, the regulatory bodies have to ensure that under-graduate medical students are trained to treat patients with knowledge as well as empathy and the medical teachers set an example in this respect for students to learn from. While the medical teacher needs to be updated on the latest medical knowledge, the ability to do medical research is not a must for imparting basic medical education. Postgraduate medical education needs teachers who are capable of managing all types of cases while imbibing new medical knowledge with the added ability to impart their knowledge to post-graduate students. An ability to do research is only an added skill that may be taught to the students. Any doctor is welcome to take up research in a full-fledged manner if he/she is so inclined but that should be the individual's choice.

Making publication of research papers mandatory for medical teachers is basically unsound. It can only 'force feed' research into those who are not inclined to it and spawn low quality and questionable research publications. It will shift the focus away from the need to train competent and compassionate doctors, which is of core importance from the point of view of a good health care system. The number of years of teaching medical students should remain *the criterion* to decide on the standing of a medical teacher, and not the number of research papers published by them. A nuanced approach by the regulatory bodies in matters of health care, medical education and research would help to avoid loss of the quality of empathy among doctors and medical students and prevent deterioration of the health care services.

References:

1. Hojat M. Ten approaches for enhancing empathy in health and human services cultures. J.Health Hum Serv Adm. 2009 Spring:31(4):412-50
http://www.ncbi.nlm.nih.gov/pubmed/19385420

2. Chen D, Lew R, Hershman W, Orlander J. A cross-sectional measurement of medical student empathy. J Gen Intern Med. 2007 Oct;22(10):1434-8. Epub 2007 Jul 26.
http://www.ncbi.nlm.nih.gov/pubmed/17653807

3. Chen DC, Kirshenbaum DS, Yan J, Kirshenbaum E, Aseltine RH Characterizing changes in student empathy throughout medical school. Med Teach. 2012:34(4):305-11.
http://www.ncbi.nlm.nih.gov/pubmed/22455699

4. Ziółkowska-Rudowicz E, Kładna A. Empathy- building of physicians (Parts I to IV). Part I--A review of applied methods Pol Merkur Lekarski. [Polish] 2010 Oct;29(172):277-81.
http://www.ncbi.nlm.nih.gov/pubmed/21207648

#12: Fixing the Basic flaw in Medical Education and Health Care

There is a basic flaw in the commonly held concept of Medicine that lies at the root of all the maladies prevailing in the field of medical education and health care. Successful practice of Medicine consists of about 2/3rd body medicine and 1/3rd mind-body and mind-body-spirit medicine. But only the 2/3rd component of body medicine is generally recognized as Medicine. The remaining 1/3rd is considered, if at all, under alternative medicine. While body medicine is based on structure and is therefore objective and easily teachable, mind-body medicine and mind-body-spirit medicine are more subjective and picked up by doctors after years of practical experience.

Medical colleges with their present curriculum can teach only the 2/3rd component; the rest of 1/3rd is mostly self-learnt by students and doctors through observation of peers and teachers who teach by setting an example. If we consider this fact it becomes obvious that too much importance is being given to activities based on something that is incomplete by itself: body medicine-based examinations, specializations, CME points, renewal of license and so on. It is appropriate to learn and update oneself about diseases of the body and their management but all such learning should be tempered by the fact that it pertains only to the 2/3rd component of Medicine. To be successfully utilized, this knowledge needs to be combined with the remaining 1/3rd component that is learnt through subjective experience. That is to say medical knowledge to be complete needs to be combined with a positive and empathetic approach towards the patient. Such a wholesome approach towards the patient not only treats the patient better but helps create better doctor-patient (or patient's attendants) relationship, avoids potential conflict and indirectly helps healing.

The incomplete and ignorant notion of Medicine that is widely prevalent not only complicates management by making its application mechanical but also results in Medicine being taught in a mechanical manner based on a curriculum that is built mainly on body medicine. The doctors thus produced, unless they are exposed to wholesome teachers, tend to behave more like machines lacking in empathy. Inappropriate glorification of body medicine encourages unnecessary investigations, escalates cost and allows third parties to take control. Instead of a wholesome approach towards patients, approaches catering to various disparate interests have come to determine medical education and health care delivery. Modern hospitals tend to become more like workshops, patients seen more as study materials and the disease burden as well as students aspiring to become doctors - fields to be harvested. Correction of the basic flaw should start with widespread recognition of the incomplete nature of grossly teachable and evaluable medicine. The Regulatory authorities should try to add completeness to medical education by emphasizing the neglected 1/3rd component of Medicine and make the wholesome medical teacher the fulcrum of all learning.

At the entry point, entrance exams to UG/PG courses should in addition to testing proficiency in the required subjects, also test the candidates' ability to feel for and render help to those in need of it. How this can be done is a matter that needs help from educationists. Mere logic-based tests in the concerned subjects as at present will only worsen the malady and chaos. Being more subtle and subjective, the 1/3rd component is easily side-lined. Corrective measures need wisdom and vision. Just as diseases like obesity, diabetes mellitus and dyslipidemia need basic life style modification to be meaningfully treated, the maladies in the field of medical education and health care require basic conceptual modification. Healing by doctors should, as a rule, imply healing of the mind, body and the spirit and not merely the body.

#13: Intuitive Medicine

In this present age of evidence-based medicine, the value of intuition in medical practice is under- rated. Generally, it is regarded with indifference if not contempt. An experienced doctor will know the importance of an intuitive approach to the patient and the patient's problem. He can differentiate between intuition and a blind guess. Delving into and understanding intuition is essential to make the best use of it [1].

What is intuition and where does this come from? From the medical stand-point, intuition can be considered to be the *feeling* within oneself about the nature of a disease or its management. It is based on one's past knowledge and experience. This knowledge or experience might have been acquired in the recent or remote past and one may not be consciously remembering as to when exactly it was acquired.

The process of acquiring knowledge may vary from being purely logical (based on evidence), to being intuitive and corroborated by the intuitive experience of others. In the present day, most of the medical knowledge in use is apparently of the first type. However, much of the knowledge we presume as being evidence-based can be shown to be intuitively acquired in the first place.

An example is the use of several drugs that are derived from herbs. For centuries, they have been used intuitively (e.g. ginger, turmeric, aloe vera) [2]. Only recently the active ingredients have been isolated and their chemical structure and mechanism of action understood. Here we see that logic has merely fine-tuned the knowledge acquired by intuition.

In fact, any new discovery is first 'intuitive' for the discoverer but later is put to test and accepted, based on 'evidence'. Intuition precedes logic. 'Knowledge' is acquired when the understanding is 'meaningful', whether by intuition or logic. The present tendency to glorify logic at the expense of intuition smothers creativity, makes the academic approach mechanical and reduces learning to mere acquisition of recorded information. At the field level, this allows medical practice to be converted into protocols that are convenient for use and can be legally and commercially exploited.

The flawed approach to academic and consequently practical medicine entails setting up of logic-based goals, while dampening intuition and freedom of the creative spirit. Curricular evaluations tend to become stereotyped and reproduction of known information accepted as evidence of learning. Inevitably, doctors are being 'produced' through a conveyor belt process where the students are made to 'learn, reproduce and forget' on their way to become 'qualified doctors'. Even practical and clinical exams tend to become stereotyped. Instead, actual work-based evaluations help encourage creative and intuitive learning.

Predominantly evidence-based medicine makes clinical practice mechanical, distancing the doctor from the patient and contributing largely to physician dis-satisfaction. Intuitively applying the knowledge one has acquired, allows creativity in clinical approach, makes it patient- friendly, ensures physician satisfaction and is cost- effective. Being open to intuitive medicine allows the seamless practice of Body medicine (that constitutes only about two-thirds of medicine) alongside Mind-Body and Mind-Body-Spirit medicine (constituting the remaining one-third of medicine) [3,4].

While logic cannot be sacrificed and there is need for basic fundamentals, medicine needs to be open-ended in theory and practice with a fine balance between logic and intuition allowing creativity at all levels. Excessive emphasis on evidence-based medicine tends to worsen the problems plaguing the field of medicine, while increased emphasis on intuitive medicine tends to simplify them. The paradigm of intuitive medicine needs to be strengthened at all levels.

References:

1. Trisha Greenhalgh. Intuition and evidence-- uneasy bedfellows? Br J Gen Pract. 2002 May;

52(478): 395–400.
https://www.ncbi.nlm.nih.gov/pmc/articles/PMC1314297/

2. Boca Raton (FL): Herbal Medicine: Biomolecular and Clinical Aspects. 2nd edition. Benzie IFF, Wachtel-Galor S, editors. CRC Press/Taylor & Francis; 2011.
https://www.ncbi.nlm.nih.gov/books/NBK92771/

3. Vijayaragh P. Becoming Aware of Mind-Body- Spirit Medicine. Future Health, Apr 2014;
http://www.futurehealth.org/articles/Becoming-Aware-of-Mind-Bod-by-Vijayaraghavan-Pad-Attitude_Body_Compassion_Comprehensive-140426-607.html

4. Vijayaragh P. Fixing the Basic Flaw in Medical Education and Health Care; Opednews, July 2016;
http://www.opednews.com/articles/Fixing-the-Basic-flaw-in-M-by-Vijayaraghavan-Pad-Doctors_Empathy_Health_Health-And-Fitness-160710-26.html

#14: Quantum View of Medicine and its Implications

The term "quantum" refers to the smallest amount of a physical quantity that can be counted or measured. The name "quantum mechanics" is derived from the observation that some physical quantities can change only in discrete amounts (Latin quanta) and not in a "continuum" way. The theory and practice of medicine needs to be understood in a similar "quantum" rather than the "continuum" way if the observed phenomena in the world of medicine are to be fully accounted for. For example, when a disease is understood to be nearly incurable by conventional medicine and is cured by an unexplained alternative medicine, this cure is usually overlooked or disregarded as an "exception." The quantum view of medicine can explain such apparent variations or exceptions.

We understand the theory of a disease (its causation and treatment) based on some scientific principles. There is a flow of logic from one aspect to the other in a continuous way as in the case of Era 1 or "body" medicine (structure-based), which constitutes most of conventional medicine. The recently understood Era 2 or "mind-body" (thought-based) and Era 3 or "mind-body-spirit" (feeling-based) medicine have their own way of understanding disease causation and treatment.[1] In practice, all these three "Eras" of medicine operate simultaneously (involving structure, thought, and feeling) in varying proportions in different individuals, with both conventional and alternative medicine having components of all three "Eras" within them.

If such a phenomenon of simultaneous working of different "Eras" is to be explained, we need to visualize medicine as consisting of "quanta" of these different "Eras." While conventional medicine is currently having Era 1 (body) as its main component with the nursing profession mainly providing the Era 2 (mind-body) and Era 3 (mind-body-spirit) components, the various streams of alternative medicine apparently have Era 2 (e.g., hypnotherapy) or Era 3 (e.g., faith healing) as their main operative component. The outcome of a disease process would be decided by the relative "quanta" of Era 1, 2, or 3 components in operation for the disease in question at the causative and therapeutic levels. The physician would use one of these "Eras" preferentially, depending on his own training and temperament.

While we see quanta of different "Eras" in operation in the same patient, each quantum will have its effect independent of what precedes, follows, or accompanies it. Medicine in real time operates in such a quantum way. This is supported by the fact that a high proportion of all patients who are treated by conventional medicine are apparently benefited by concomitant use of some form of alternative medicine.[2] The Era 2 and Era 3 components in the different forms of alternative medicine apparently contribute substantially to their unexplained effectiveness.

There is need for a common coherent model to understand and assimilate the different philosophical approaches of conventional and alternative medicine.[3] The quantum view of medicine, by understanding conventional and alternative medicine in terms of the three "Eras," gives a meaningful basis to comprehend all three. It paves the way for a system that values the individual doctor's subjective experience in treating patients on par with acquisition of scientific knowledge in the concerned field. It provides a common platform for teaching and learning all three "Eras" -- the body, mind-body, and mind-body-spirit components of medicine. It allows the inclusion of positive thoughts and an empathetic attitude toward the patient as integral parts of therapy.

References:

1. Padmanabhan V. Becoming Aware of Mind-Body- Spirit Medicine; 2014. Available from: http://www.futurehealth.org/articles/Becoming-Aware-of-Mind-Bod-by-Vijayaraghavan-Pad-

Attitude_Body_Compassion_Comprehensive-140426-607.html.

2. The Use of Complementary and Alternative Medicine in the United States. Available from: https://nccih.nih.gov/research/statistics/2007/camsurvey_fs1.htm.

3. FDA and the Challenge of Alternative Medicine: Realistic Assessments and Regulatory Flexibility. Available from: https://dash.harvard.edu/bitstream/handle/1/8852106/Tricia_M_Hwang.pdf?sequence=1

#15: The Need for Empathy-Based Medical Education

The Medical Council of India has recently released the document titled *Competency Based Undergraduate Curriculum for The Indian Medical Graduate* (2018).[1] It has been officially announced that the new curriculum will be introduced for the MBBS students from the academic year 2019–2020. It seeks to replace the existing curriculum, which was notified in 1997.

Competency is the central theme in the document. The competencies to be acquired by the student are divided into general competencies and sub-competencies (or subject-wise competencies). Under the latter, there are 23 subjects (including preclinical, paraclinical, medicine and allied, and surgery and allied subjects). Under these, there are 412 topics, and under these, 2949 competencies are to be taught during the entire curriculum.

The new curriculum has a separate module called AETCOM – Attitude, Ethics, and Communication competencies,[2] giving due importance to the crucial aspect of developing the right attitude toward the patient. Learning modules for AETCOM are spread over all the 4 years and are rightly planned to be implemented first.

While the AETCOM competencies have empathetic consideration of the patient as the base, there are enough reasons to move toward a full-fledged empathy-based medical curriculum. There has been worldwide attention to the central role of empathy in medical education.[3] The basic premise of the medical profession has empathy toward those suffering from some ailment. The basic reason why students (most, if not all) opt for the medical profession is the motivation to cure patients. However, there is realization that the process of medical education itself leads to loss of empathy since students are trained for the "left brain-dominant, linear, stepwise, analytical, and evidence-based knowledge." Screening humanistic qualities (altruism, compassion) and assessing the Student's emotional intelligence quotient during the medical admission selection process have been mooted to ensure the quality of empathy in the would-be doctors.[4]

The value of empathy is taught implicitly, through personal example, by a physician during interactions with the patients. The manner in which the physician listens to the patient and addresses his/her concerns leaves an impression on the students who accompany him/her during rounds. Students who are empathetic by nature preserve and foster their own quality of empathy by seeing their teachers as role models.

The precious quality of empathy needs to be directed toward areas of patient care that the student finds to be intellectually interesting. Although the medical student needs to acquire various competencies in different subjects appropriate to the times, he or she should be given the opportunity to acquire the needed competencies in the subject that kindles his or her interest. Disregarding this self-determined interest, if the student is made to learn competencies as per a fixed schedule, it would not be conducive to the preservation and expression of the quality of empathy.

Taking a quantum view of medicine is a simple way of integrating the quality of empathy within the curriculum. Here, conventional medicine (with aspects of alternative medicine) is considered to have the components of body medicine, mind–body medicine, and mind–body–spirit medicine, which are understood to act simultaneously and independent of one another. Students can express the quality of empathy without compromising the academic approach for understanding and practice of medicine.[5]

There is need for considering the development of an empathy-based curriculum that allows the self-determined interest of students to express itself and avoids the rigorous expectations of a competence-based curriculum.

References:

1. Medical Council of India. Competency Based Undergraduate Curriculum for The Indian Medical Graduate. Vol. 1. Medical Council of India; 2018. https://www.old.mciindia.org/UG-Curriculum/UG-Curriculum-Vol-I.pdf.
2. Medical Council of India: AETCOM Competencies for Indian Medical Graduate. https://www.old.mciindia.org/UG-Curriculum/AETCOM_book.pdf.
3. Pedersen R. Empathy development in medical education – A critical review. Med Teach 2010;32:593-600.
4. Shelley BP. A value forgotten in doctoring: Empathy. Arch Med Health Sci 2015;3:169- 73.
5. Vijayaraghavan P. Quantum view of medicine and its implications. Int J Acad Med 2017;3:334-5. http://www.ijam-web.org/article.asp?issn=2455-5568;year=2017;volume=3;issue=2;spage=334;epage=335;aulast=Vijayaraghavan.

#16: Halting Dehumanization in Medicine

Introduction:
The process of dehumanization in medicine is a cause of concern for everyone. The subject has been discussed from a psychological perspective by Haque and Waytz,[1] covering primarily the dehumanization related to doctor–patient relationship. However, the process of dehumanization extends beyond this and affects the whole health-care system. Dehumanization affects the physician himself who has become more of a doctor-machine. The constant expansion of medical information and the compulsion to remain in touch with evidence-based updates, takes the physician away from the patient. The analytic and objective outlook that is required separates the physician from his/her own source of inner joy. To address these concerns, the roots of health and disease as well as the process of dehumanization need to be understood from a deeper mind–body–spirit perspective.

Dimensions of Health and Disease:
Recent advances have established that the health of an individual depends not merely on body health but also on the health of the mind (local and personal) and the spirit (non-local and transpersonal). Medicine may be considered to have three coexisting

and overlapping eras: Era I or body medicine, Era II or mind-body medicine and Era III or mind-body-spirit medicine.[2],[3] As per the "quantum view of medicine," therapy in medicine is understood to consist of "quanta" or independent and simultaneously operating components of body medicine (structure-based), mind–body medicine (thought-based), and mind–body–spirit medicine (feeling-based).[4] The practice of medicine with the awareness of the "quanta" within a therapy (quantum-aware approach) is holistic.

Physician's Health:
The physician, being the agent of therapy to the patient, is human and dependent on his/her own state of health. The physician, just as any other individual, needs to be healthy for being efficient and productive. Conventional medicine has apparently developed excess of body medicine with neglect of the mind–body and mind–body–spirit aspects of medicine. It is appropriate for a medical student, as a beginner, to consider primarily the bodily aspect of disease with the application of the faculty of objective thinking. While communication skills (pertaining to mind and spirit) are recognized to be an important part of medical training,[5] in actual practice, they tend to be neglected because there is little requirement for empathy and a persistent demand for the use of the analytic mind in conventional body medicine. In the absence of a

functional framework that allows balanced use of all the three components, imbalance in the physician's own health results, leaving many physicians emotionally and spiritually deprived (physician "burnout").[6]

Evidence-Based Body Medicine is Downstream: The near-exclusive development of body medicine, without recognition of the other two components, has resulted in interpreting every disease in terms of structural derangement, while the origin of the disease could well be in the mental and spiritual dimensions. It is found that changes in the latter two dimensions result in structural changes at the genetic and consequently the molecular level in animal studies as well as in postmortem human brain.[7] A sedentary behavior (alteration in mental and spiritual dimensions) resulting in diabetes mellitus (effect in the body dimension) is another example. Tackling only the elevated blood sugar amounts to intervening at a lower level when the behavioral cause is upstream. The constant expansion of medical knowledge needs to be considered in this context of viewing the pathogenesis of every disease as a structural derangement. Understanding of a disease down to the genomic level does not alter the primary truth upstream. The expansion of such analytic and evidence-based medicine tends to keep the physician away from the core of the patient's problem.

Humans Perform Better with Intuitive rather than Logical Approach:
By evolution, the human brain is better in choosing from probabilities (intuitive) rather than working with certitude (logic). Learning from prior experience is more efficacious.[8],[9] Moreover, intuitive approach, which is creative and fundamental to hypothesis generation,[10] can reach the core of the patient's concern with ease, but has become neglected. When the physician's work is predominantly objective and evidence-based, it is out of tune with his/her inborn faculties of being creative and intuitive, thus cutting him/her off from a source of joy and contributing to increased stress.

Putting Empathetic Understanding before Evidence-Based Consideration:
The "quantum-aware" approach toward the patient, by allowing an empathetic connection, results in simultaneous objective and subjective understanding of the patient's problem covering all the three dimensions. For example, the ideal management of a case of diabetes mellitus would include not only advice on calorie restriction and use of hypoglycemic agents (body aspect), but also an understanding of the patient's behavioral circumstances (mental and spiritual aspects) that

may require modifications. Such a multidimensional approach comes instinctively for the physician who is connected empathetically with the patient. By suggesting suitable lifestyle modifications, the physician does what is most appropriate for the patient. He/she does this more out of empathetic connection than from mere evidence-based consideration. The physician does "objectify the patient" to facilitate clinical problem solving, but awareness of the "mind–body–spirit" component avoids dehumanization of the patient and at the same time gives satisfaction to the physician as well as the patient.

Direct Experience with Patients Helps Develop Quantum Awareness:
Developing the holistic "quantum-aware" approach in clinical medicine requires the physician to have a sound, but not necessarily a constantly updated knowledge of conventional body medicine. More importantly, it requires a positive approach and empathy toward the patient, covering the mental and spiritual dimensions. As the development of quantum-awareness is proportional to direct experience with patients, working with patients is just as important for the clinician as acquiring theoretical updates on the bodily aspect of diseases. A few more minutes of the physician's time applied purposefully, would change the conventional objective approach into the holistic "quantum-

aware" approach. Beyond the patient, adopting the "quantum-aware" approach as a standard practice among clinicians has significant implications for the entire health-care system.

Balanced Use of Resources:
Scientific advances in body medicine, though evidence-based, are infructuous unless they are meaningfully applied. "To cure sometimes, to relieve often, to comfort always" are words of medical wisdom. Situations such as inappropriate availability of high-tech medical equipment in the face of neglect of basic patient care, result from overemphasis on body medicine, which is virtually taken to be the sole aspect of medicine.[11] The attitude of "quantum-aware" approach leads to a balanced consideration of all the three components and a meaningful use of resources.

Recognizing the Value of Physician's Experience:
In the field of medical education, the apparently logical need for remaining updated with advances in body medicine will be tempered by the importance of considering health and disease in all the three dimensions. The physician who has developed a balanced outlook to all the three components through years of practice, is an asset. To consider disqualifying a physician simply because he/she is not updated with the latest in body medicine, will not

be tenable when its constantly expanding downstream nature is recognized.

Conclusion:
Predominant application of evidence-based body medicine with neglect of mind–body and mind–body–spirit aspects has led to a pervasive dehumanizing effect involving the patient, the physician, health-care delivery, and medical education. The "quantum-aware" approach, where there is balanced consideration of all the three components, allows the physician to be competent, intuitive, creative, and empathetic, being capable of reaching the core of the patient's concern. Health-care delivery and the process of medical education are modified accordingly. In short, while medicine is learned from the "head," it needs to be applied from the "heart" to halt the process of dehumanization in medicine.

References:

1. Haque OS, Waytz A. Dehumanization in medicine: Causes, solutions, and functions. Perspect Psychol Sci 2012;7:176-86.

2. Seaward BL. Stress and human spirituality 2000: At the cross roads of physics and metaphysics. Appl Psychophysiol Biofeedback

2000;25:241-6.

3. Larry Dossey. A Conversation about the Future of Medicine. Available from: http://www.dosseydossey.com/larry/QnA.html

4. Vijayaraghavan P. Quantum view of medicine and its implications. Int J Acad Med 2017;3:334. Available from: http://www.ijam-web.org/text.asp?2017/3/2/334/222480

5. Choudhary A, Gupta V. Teaching communications skills to medical students: Introducing the fine art of medical practice. Int J Appl Basic Med Res 2015;5:S41-4.

6. Drummond D. Physician burnout: Its origin, symptoms, and five main causes. Fam Pract Manag 2015;22:42-7.

7. How Stress can Change your DNA. SITN, Nov 2017. Harvard University. Available from: http://sitn.hms.harvard.edu/flash/2017/stress-induced-dna-modification-may-play-role-mentalillness/

8. Laura Sanders. The Probabilistic Mind. Science News; October, 2011. Available from: https://lightdark.org/s/GirshickScienceNewsProbabilistic-mind.pdf

9. Gigerenzer G. Gut Feelings. The Intelligence of the Unconscious; 2007. Available from: https://www.mpib-berlin.mpg.de/en/research/adaptive-behavior-andcognition/publications/books/gut-feelings

10. Greenhalgh T. Intuition and evidence-uneasy bedfellows? Br J Gen Pract 2002;52:395-400.

11. High Tech Medicine Can Be Bad for Your Health. Allen Frances, HuffPost; October, 2015. Available from: https://www.huffpost.com/entry/high-tech-medicine-can-be_b_8331406?guccounter=1&guce_referrer=aHR0cHM6Ly93d3cuZ29vZ2xlLmNvbS8&guce_referrer_sig=AQAAAG01TMJOda0IqC2O%20BgssNxQNuMpemwctUhMz-%20ASWDTu6-mkb9_kqbNvtCCCiGSI4obWTRPHhYy1Kpp95I qmKhYAv4S_HOIZ7zLJSsJBsrvU6S4zn6noSVp eF2I5ak%203fxWCF7iDpCJWkp%20TH3SM7C aehXnK_isSuOnQ%204A38bmcQCbi

#17: Connecting with Spiritual Intelligence in Medicine

Introduction:
With ever-increasing medical knowledge, remaining updated within one's area of work is a challenging task. The problem is compounded even more in these pandemic times. Technological innovations have been playing an increasing role in the practice of medicine. Applications such as artificial intelligence may help in making faster diagnoses of the structural (body) aspects of diseases, but every disease also has thought-based (mind) and feeling-based (spirit) components that are beyond the realm of the machine.[1],[2] In this context, it is appropriate to remind ourselves of spiritual intelligence (SQ), the hidden tool that is within each one of us.

The Three inner Faculties:
When the disease is new with no existing protocols or if the protocols are changing frequently because of new developments, the clinician may come up with a novel way of treating the disease based on past experiences and direct observations. In fact, this is how new treatment methods are developed, which are then corroborated by similar methods developed by others. The astute clinician instinctively tries a new treatment in an urgent situation, which turns out to be successful. This

aspect of the physician has been at the forefront during these uncertain days of the COVID-19 pandemic.

Treatment based on existing concepts and available protocols requires prior knowledge and is based on cognitive intelligence or intelligence quotient (IQ).
Applying the knowledge appropriately to the patient requires an empathetic connection with the patient and is based on emotional intelligence or emotional quotient (EQ). Coming up with a concept or treatment that is completely new and yet suitable for a clinical situation requires not only background knowledge and an empathetic connection with the patient (IQ and EQ) but also a connection with the physician's own creative "inner self" or "soul," which is spiritual intelligence or SQ (Spiritual Quotient). While IQ is logical and EQ is intuitive, SQ is instinctive. The instinctive wisdom of SQ is not the exclusive territory of the astute clinician. Every one of us has all these three faculties, but formal learning and practice of medicine have hitherto been mainly IQ and EQ based.[3]

Integrating Aspect of SQ:
The "inner self" or "soul" is pure consciousness that is reached by each one of us during the stage of deep sleep. The information and experiences of the waking state are presumably integrated and made meaningful during the bliss of deep sleep. This is the

integrating aspect of SQ, which is inbuilt. After the person wakes up, the blissful wisdom of deep sleep is carried forward, informing and influencing the thoughts and actions of the day. A shortfall in the quality of deep sleep is reflected as lack of bliss and an impaired SQ.

Expressive Aspect of SQ:
Spiritual intelligence is by nature comfortable with positive human qualities such as truth, love, and peace. If these qualities are lacking, the "inner self" is not satisfied giving rise to unease or stress experienced by the individual. SQ (relating to the "inner self" or "soul") is the base from which IQ and EQ (relating to "self" or ego) operate during the waking state. The individual connected with the "inner self" is calm, composed, and gives his (or her) best. Such an individual can function from the level of "self" or ego as well as from "inner self." Recently, studies in neuroscience have clarified how IQ, EQ, and SQ work and are related to each other. While IQ pertains to the left brain and EQ to the right brain, SQ involves synchronous activity of the whole brain.[4]

Good Quality Clinical Work Depends on Finely balanced IQ and EQ:
Clinical work involving patients helps to fine-tune the EQ of the physician. On the other hand, when fascination for acquiring knowledge leads to

overemphasis on IQ, neglect of EQ can result.[5] What matters is a fine balance between IQ and EQ, functioning on the base of a sound SQ, for optimal performance. This applies not only to health professionals but also to all individuals.

Meeting the Challenge of Dealing with Uncertainties:
Physicians may tend to become biased in favor of using either their IQ or EQ. Especially in critical situations, they may tend to become either too objective or too subjective. However, the physician who is calm and connected to his "inner self," uses the instinctive wisdom of his SQ by maintaining a balance between IQ and EQ and bringing the best out of these two faculties. He will be comfortable in dealing with uncertainties at a time when tolerating uncertainty has become a challenge for the health care system.[6] He can navigate through any clinical situation with confidence and equanimity. In addition, the process of becoming updated with the latest knowledge becomes a creative and selective process. The physician instinctively chooses what is relevant and meaningful from a plethora of available information.

Tapping the Potential of the Soul:
In recent times, the importance of being connected with the "soul" is being increasingly recognized in every field of activity.[7] The practice of meditation

helps to gain awareness and connection with one's "inner self" or "soul." The process and the beneficial effects of meditation have been well studied.[8] While everyone benefits by practicing meditation and connecting with the "soul," it is relevant to note that the quality of work of the physician is also enhanced. With awareness of the "inner self" comes the ability to move between the ego and the "soul."[9] When the development of this ability forms the core of medical education, it allows the full potential of the physician as a human resource to be tapped and utilized.

Conclusion:
Connecting with SQ or the "inner self" or "soul" can be a simple and natural process for some but can be strange and difficult for many, since matters pertaining to the "soul" have become neglected in this age of science and technology. Individual insights corroborated by studies in neuroscience have simplified its understanding bringing it within the grasp of the modern mind. The instinctive wisdom of SQ can be utilized by the individual when there is a fine balance between IQ and EQ. While connecting with SQ benefits everyone, it is of particular relevance for the physician in patient care as well as in medical education. Of even more significance is that whenever the hidden tool of SQ is utilized, physicians as human beings enjoy fulfillment and peace within.

References:

1. Amisha, Malik P, Pathania M, Rathaur VK. Overview of artificial intelligence in medicine. J Family Med Prim Care. 2019;8:2328-31. doi:10.4103/jfmpc.jfmpc_440_19.

2. Vijayaraghavan P. Quantum view of medicine and its implications. Int J Acad Med 2017;3:334-5.

3. Moawad H. How Physicians Can Develop EQ; 2018. Available from: https://www.hcplive.com/view/how-physicians-can-develop-eq.

4. Griffiths R. Top Ten Features of Spiritual Intelligence; 2014-2019. Available from: https://sqi.co/top-ten-features-spiritual-intelligence/.

5. Is IQ overrated in Medicine? Advisory Board; 2018. Available from: https://www.advisory.com/daily-briefing/2018/02/14/emotional-intelligence. [Last accessed on 2021 Feb 21].

6. Simpkin AL, Schwartzstein RM. Tolerating uncertainty – The next medical revolution? N Engl J Med 2016;375:1713-5.

7. Snowise K. 3 Ways to Deepen the Connection with your Soul-Self. HuffPost; 2016. Available from: https://www.huffpost.com/entry/3-ways-to-deepen-the-conn_b_8905658.

8. Sharma H. Meditation: Process and effects. Ayu 2015;36:233-7.

9. Rios J. How to Move from Ego to Soul: Spiritual Intelligence; 2017. Available from: https://www.findhorn.org/front-page/spiritual-intelligence/.

#18: Consciousness as the Basis of Disease and Disaster

Introduction: The process of seeking the meaning of any new situation can open up unforeseen insight and understanding. The scale of disruption caused by Covid-19 pandemic prompted many to seek a meaning for the crisis that has impacted the world, much beyond the conventional realm of public health. The phrase 'everything is interconnected' is well exemplified by the widespread consequences of the pandemic and the measures needed to overcome them. As the pandemic is being brought under control, there is outbreak of war in Ukraine that is threatening to spread to other nations. We also have the climate crisis, which is slowly and surely endangering the world. These and several other crises affecting the world one after another, may be viewed as unconnected events, but as physicians trained to go into the root cause of anything that affects the health of human beings, one can perceive shifts in consciousness as the common basis underlying them, through inquiry and introspection.

Taking the intuitive view: Though humans perceive events and understand them based on logic, the cognition usually starts as intuition and logic comes thereafter. Intuition can have as its basis, past experiences that may or may not be remembered.[1] Two intuitive theories of causation concerning human nature, the theory of imbalance of human tendencies and the theory of karma, throw light on the possible chain of events leading to the occurrence of diseases and disasters in general. Before going into these intuitive theories of causation and how they involve shifts in consciousness, the first question that needs an answer is: how does the perceived shift in consciousness translate into, in the case of Covid-19, the structure and function of the virus and its variants that apparently cause the havoc?

The common basis of consciousness and its equilibrium: Empirically there is evidence that the consciousness (awareness) underlying human nature and behavior, is the basis of health and disease.[2] Taking a larger perspective, consciousness can be considered to be the basis of everything in the universe (panpsychism),[3] including the myriad living and non-living entities, which are thus inexplicably interconnected. Diseases and disasters, explained through various theories of causation, involve shifts in consciousness. They are resolved when there is corrective change, which presumably maintains the individual and collectively, the universal consciousness [known in Yoga as *Sat-chit-ananda* [4] (truth-consciousness-bliss)], in equilibrium. Implied in this concept of universal consciousness is the philosophical assumption that consciousness preceded and is hence the basis of the entire universe.

Theory of imbalance of human tendencies: According to the first of the two intuitive theories of causation, any disease is said to be a manifestation of imbalance of tendencies or *Gunas* [5] present in every individual. The health of individuals depends on a fine balance between three in-born tendencies viz. active, passive and the serene. Active tendency leads to a dominant mindset, passive tendency to inertia and attachment, while the serene tendency enlightens and uniquely heals the disturbances arising from the first two. When there is an imbalance between the three tendencies, disease manifests in the individual. The process of undergoing the disease serves to restore the balance between the tendencies.

Extrapolating this concept, a global imbalance of the three tendencies might have predisposed the human society to the pandemic. A violent mindset (active) and excessive sensory attachments (passive) were rampant, and the serene tendency subdued, in the pre-Covid times. Faced with the Covid-19 calamity, the instinct for survival may be forcing a change in human behavior and we may be seeing signs of dampening of the active and passive tendencies, and a corresponding augmentation of the serene tendency. The value of being serene and allowing health appropriate behavior to become central to life, instead of allowing unrestrained active and passive tendencies, is being learnt the hard way. If this is so, then one can expect the pandemic to go on until the global imbalance of human tendencies is largely set right.

Theory of karma: Karma [6] refers to the principle of cause and effect where one's thoughts and actions determine the course of one's life, good action leading to good result and bad action resulting in bad result. The karmic principle applied to the world at large, intuitively throws light on the cause of the present situation and the possible future course of events. Now, the following key question arises - how is karma determined to be good or bad?

The karmic principle can be rationalized based on the concept of 'self' and 'Self' (or 'inner self'). The 'Self' is 'pure consciousness', whose nature is 'truth-consciousness-bliss' or *Sat-chit-ananda*, identical with universal consciousness mentioned earlier. The 'self' (or ego) is what we perceive of ourselves in the waking state. The 'Self' is blissful by itself and is reached by every individual subconsciously during the state of deep sleep. When the thoughts and actions of the 'self' is in tune with the 'truth-consciousness-bliss' nature of the 'Self' within, the individuals are at peace with themselves; harmony prevails in all spheres of activity and the karma that accumulates from such activity is good. When the 'self' is in conflict with the 'Self' within, the thoughts and actions of individuals go against 'truth-consciousness-bliss' and bad karma builds up. The individual, and by extension the society, has to undergo the consequences of accumulated good and bad karma.

It is a fact that in recent times, much of the collective human thoughts and actions have been out of tune with 'truth-consciousness-bliss' nature of 'Self', which is expressed rather simplistically but succinctly as the 'seven social sins'.[7] The consequences of accumulated bad karma are possibly manifesting as the pandemic, a war that threatens to become global, an imminent disastrous climate change and so on.

Restoring the equilibrium of consciousness: However, mankind can endure and overcome these adverse situations through augmentation of the serene tendency that allows it to attune itself back with the 'truth-consciousness-bliss' nature of the 'Self', accumulate good karma and help hasten the end of the pandemic. An active or passive tendency that is preoccupied with the 'self' and keeps away from the 'Self', predisposes to bad karma and perpetuates the adversity. A disastrous climate change or a global war between nations may become nature's way of dealing with the problem in a 'surgical' way, when a 'medical' way like Covid-19 pandemic proves to be insufficient. Human behavioral change is the means, for reaching the goal of restoration of equilibrium of individual and collective consciousness.

Conclusion: It is useful and instructive to view diseases and disasters as shifts in consciousness, from both the individual as well as collective points of view. Dwelling and acting upon the 'Self' ('inner self' or pure consciousness) within, instead of being carried away by one's 'self' or ego, through augmentation of the serene tendency, is a behavioral change every individual can make through practice. This will hasten the resolution of diseases and disasters, both at the individual and collective levels. Insight into the role of consciousness offers a new dimension to the understanding of pathogenesis and management of diseases and disasters.

References:

[1] Rich Gasaway. (2020) Where does intuition come from. Situational Awareness Matters. Available from: www.samatters.com/intuition-come/

[2] Vijayaraghavan Padmanabhan. (2011) When consciousness becomes the basis of structure.

Available from:
https://futurehealth.org/articles/When-Consciousness-Becomes-by-Vijayaraghavan-Pad-101205-466.html

[3] Gareth Cook. (2020) Does consciousness pervade the universe? Scientific American. Available from: www.scientificamerican.com/article/does-consciousness-pervade-the-universe/

[4] Sat-chit-ananda. (2019) Yogapedia. Available from: www.yogapedia.com/definition/5838/sat-chit-ananda

[5] Timothy Burgin. (2019) The 3 Gunas of Nature. Yogabasics.com Available from: www.yogabasics.com/learn/the-3-gunas-of-nature/

[6] Karma. Britannica. Available from: https://www.britannica.com/topic/karma

[7] Seven Social Sins. Wikipedia. Available from: https://en.wikipedia.org/wiki/Seven_Social_Sins

#19: A common platform for all systems of medicine

Introduction: Those trained in conventional scientific medicine find it difficult to come to terms with the alternative systems of medicine [1]. Conventional scientific medicine, also called Allopathy, is based on an understanding of medicine in terms of physics, chemistry, biology and maths. In addition, an understanding of the emotional and behavioural aspects of human beings helps in the successful practice of medicine.

Recently, because of their acclaimed usefulness, alternative systems of medicine including Acupuncture, Hypnotherapy and what is known in India as AYUSH (Ayurveda, Yoga & Naturopathy, Unani, Siddha, Homeopathy), are being increasingly accepted [2]. Practitioners of conventional medicine may accept the use of alternative systems as long as they are not harmful to the patient from the scientific point of view. But these complementary systems of medicine are nevertheless kept at a distance, since they do not make sense to the scientifically trained mind, in spite of empirical studies supporting their effectiveness.

In 1993 the US Congress decided that America should take a more scientific look at alternative medicine and established within the Office of the Director of the National Institutes of Health (NIH) the Office of Alternative Medicine (OAM). The FDA, the regulatory body in USA for granting recognition to treatment modalities, was expected to address this issue meaningfully but a coherent understanding about alternative systems of medicine [3] still remains elusive. This situation, in spite of the popularity and perceived effectiveness of the alternative systems, has led either to their reluctant acceptance or total rejection by the scientific community.

In India, Ayurveda, Siddha and Unani have been used successfully for the past several centuries and have become part of culture. As per CRMI (Compulsory Rotating Medical 178 Internship) regulations 2021 of the NMC (National Medical Commission), 7 days of AYUSH posting has been included within the one-year internship from 2022-23 [4]. Now, the UG medical (MBBS) student is faced with the situation of remaining in a state of denial or accepting alternate systems unquestioningly much against the scientific temper that is essential for practicing conventional medicine. In such a situation, a common platform for comprehending conventional as well as alternate systems of medicine has become more relevant.

The common platform: What is it that is common to all systems of medicine? Alternative systems have theories that do not fit into the basics of conventional medicine. However, every system of medicine can be found to address three components of patient care viz. body, mind and spirit. While managing any medical condition, these three components respectively target the structure (body), influence the thought (mind) and connect with the feeling (spirit) of the patient in varying proportions.

The three components in conventional medicine: Conventional medicine, until recently, was considered to address only the structural aspect but has now been shown to address all the three components. The evolution of modern medicine can be divided into three eras: – Era 1: Body Medicine, Era 2: Mind-Body Medicine, Era 3: Mind-Body-Spirit Medicine [5].

Era 1, since the 1860s, is plain old mechanical medicine. The body is not functioning properly, so the 'doctor-mechanic' uses whatever tools of treatment are available to fix the problem. Era 2 medicine since the 1940s, was initially about psycho-somatic diseases, arising from negative thoughts. It is today called 'Mind-Body medicine', which is basically about the impact of thought, feeling and belief, within an individual. Era 3 Medicine, since the 1990s, is based upon the ability of the mind to function trans-personally or non-locally. That is to say, the ability of the mind to function beyond the individual. This is supported by two bodies of evidence: Prayer, and Transpersonal imagery.

1) Prayer: It was noted that some people got well even though no medical treatment was given, except prayer. In a 1988 controlled study in San Francisco General Hospital (as well as in hundreds of similar studies), the group that was prayed for appeared to do much better than the group which received no prayer. *2) Transpersonal imagery:* It has been showed that 179 people who hold positive images of a distant person, in a way that is caring, compassionate and prayer-like, can actually bring about physical changes in that distant person.

Prayer and 'prayerfulness' have as their central feature, empathy for the subject prayed for. They display non-local manifestations of consciousness. There is another aspect of mind- body-spirit medicine that depends on the physician's empathy, acting from within the patient. Faith developed by the patient through the healing words of the physician, is its basis. Faith is a deep-seated feeling that leads to contentment and soothes the questioning mind. An empathetic approach by the physician helps the patient develop faith. Without faith the mind is active and restless. This has repercussions on the immune system, a fact that has been validated by several studies in the field of psychoneuroimmunology [6].

Taking the quantum view: Having made sense

about the scientific basis for Era 2 and Era 3 components pertaining to conventional medicine, there is need to comprehend how exactly the three components act together to benefit the patient. Each of these Era 1, Era 2 and Era 3 components can be viewed as 'quanta' of different eras. The term 'quantum' refers to the smallest amount of a physical quantity that can change only in discrete amounts and not in a 'continuum' way.

For example, we often see a disease that is difficult to manage by conventional medicine but is successfully treated by the additional use of an alternative medicine, as in using Hypnotherapy in addition to drugs for the treatment of Bronchial Asthma [7]. Here we see 'quanta' of different 'Eras' (Era 1 and Era 2) acting simultaneously on the same patient, with each 'quantum' having its effect independent of what accompanies it. Medicine in real time operates in such a 'quantum' way, rather than in a 'continuum' way that excludes additional influences.

Conventional medicine is currently having Era 1 (body) as its main component, with the nursing profession mainly providing the Era 2 (mind-body) and Era 3 (mind-body-spirit) components. The various streams of alternative medicine possibly have an Era 1 component, which is more intuitive than scientific, while Era 2 (e.g., hypnotherapy) or Era 3 (e.g., faith healing) may be their main operative component.

Conclusion: For students of conventional medicine, some familiarity with the theory concerning the 'body' component of alternative systems will suffice, since the 'mind' and 'spirit' components are common to all. Understanding patient care in terms of the three components or 'quanta' gives a common platform to make sense of all systems of medicine. Finally, taking a 'quantum view of medicine' encourages a more purposeful and balanced use of all the three components by every practitioner of medicine.

References:

[1] List of forms of alternative medicine. Wikipedia. Available from: https://en.wikipedia.org/wiki/List_of_forms_of_alternative_medicine

[2] The role of complementary and alternative medicine. E Ernst. BMJ 2000 Nov 4; 321(7269): 1133–1135. DOI: 10.1136/bmj.321.7269.1133

[3] Tricia M Hwang. FDA and the Challenge of Alternative Medicine: Realistic Assessments and Regulatory Flexibility. 1997. Available from: https://dash.harvard.edu/bitstream/handle/1/8852106/Tricia_M_Hwang.pdf?sequence=1

[4] 7 days AYUSH internship to stay for MBBS students. Medical Dialogues, Dec 2022. Available from: https://medicaldialogues.in/health-news/nmc/7-days-ayush-internshipto-stay-for-mbbs-students-85416

[5] Larry Dossey. A Conversation About the Future of Medicine. Reinventing Medicine, 2000. Available from: https://www.equilibrium-e3.com/images/PDF/A%20Conversation%20About%20the%20Future%20of%20Medicine%20with%20Larry%20Dosey.pdf

[6] Vijayaraghavan P. Improving the quality of health from within. Futurehealth.org 2012. Available from: https://www.futurehealth.org/populum/page.php?f=Improving-the- Quality-of-H-by-Vijayaraghavan-Pad-110501-893.html

[7] T C Ewer, D E Stewart Improvement in bronchial hyper-responsiveness in patients with moderate asthma after treatment with a hypnotic technique: a randomized control trial. BMJ (Clin Res Ed). 1986 Nov 1;293(6555):1129-32. DOI: 10.1136/bmj.293.6555.1129

#20: Clarity as against Certainty in Medicine

Introduction: Clarity and Certainty, though synonyms, are not exactly the same. While understanding phenomena, and especially during the practice of medicine, both clarity and certainty play crucial roles. Though clarity and certainty are intertwined, there is a subtle difference between the two and in the way they impact the course of events.

Origin of Clarity and Certainty: Clarity implies something that is clear, while certainty implies something that is backed by evidence. Though clarity and certainty are felt by the human being, both these perceptions have different origins. Clarity is felt deep within one's being or consciousness, arises from being connected with the 'pure consciousness' of one's 'inner self' and can be cultivated through meditation (Sharma, 2015). Certainty is felt based on facts and is perceived by the mind. Clarity is subjectively felt, revealing and satisfying, while certainty is more objective and based on reasoning.

The apparently limitless wisdom of 'pure consciousness': The 'pure consciousness' of 'inner self' is reached by every individual in the deep sleep state (although subconsciously) and is felt as blissful clarity on reaching the waking state. Conversely, the individual experiencing clarity can be presumed to be connected with the limitless wisdom of 'pure consciousness' of 'inner self'. It has been shown that the subconscious 'inner self' is the base for SQ or 'spiritual intelligence', from which EQ or 'emotional intelligence' and IQ or 'cognitive intelligence' arise in the waking state (Padmanabhan, 2021).

Eclipsing of Clarity: While objective certainty can contribute to subjective clarity, certainty pertains to and is limited by the logic of the mind. Clarity is beyond the mind, pertaining to consciousness. However, seeking a sense of mooring, the mind is attracted towards certainty of logic in whatever that is perceived; subjective clarity sounds inadequate and may be considered as lacking in scientific rigor. The eclipsing of clarity by the certainty of logic has deep implications (Kamaraj, 2021), that apply also for the practice of medicine.

Impact on practice of medicine: Medicine has progressed and worked wonders by focusing on the clarity of concepts rather than on certainty of facts. Measuring blood pressure with the mercury manometer and the BP cuff is a rough estimate, but still has been widely and successfully used because of the conceptual clarity it has provided. Innumerable drugs, which are plant derivatives, have been discovered instinctively and used for hundreds of years based on clarity regarding their gross action. However, further advances like elucidation of their molecular structure and mechanism of action have served to fine-tune their usefulness (Ciddi Veeresham, 2012). In recent times, with the exception of narrative medicine (Kim Krisberg, 2017), the tendency to seek objective certainty has been largely driving advances in medicine. The reductionist approach of making distinctions on ever-narrower grounds has become a logical and fascinating compulsion, contributing to the increasing complexity of modern medicine (Paul, 2001). Because of the predilection for objectivity, the simple and subtle truths perceived by the clinician have come to be ignored on the grounds of being subjective. While it is widely acknowledged that medicine is a science as well as an art, the objectivity of the science invariably pushes behind the subjectivity of the art (Hamish, 2000).

The need for a simple approach in patient care: The increasing complexity in medicine has strained patient care, which basically needs to consider the patient as a whole and not as a sum of parts. There needs to be an acceptable method that embraces the complexity arising from objectivity and yet provide a simple basis to provide wholesome care. Recently, the concept of 'complex adaptive systems' (Joachim, 2009) that seeks to accommodate unknown factors and changing clinical circumstances, has emerged in the quest towards this goal. In this regard, clarity perceived within the physician, can be considered to be a 'complex adaptive system', that has the potential to provide a simple basis for taking optimal decisions in complex situations.

Clarity allows heuristic approach: In other words, by prioritizing clarity over certainty, we have the heuristic approach (How heuristic thinking helps in reasoning logically, 2020), the common-sense approach that is widely used. Spiritual intelligence is at work when common sense is instinctively used along with clarity. The heuristic approach is at ease with uncertainty and is better suited than an algorithmic approach under changing clinical conditions.It considers the objective and the subjective perceptions without bias and facilitates good-enough decisions to be made within a limited time frame.

Conclusion: There is need to become aware of the profound value of clarity in the field of medicine. Objective certainty may help development of clarity but it may be prudent if it is not sought in everything. Routinely seeking and applying certainty within medicine expands objective knowledge and increases the complexity of medicine.

References:

- Ciddi Veeresham. Natural products derived from plants as a source of drugs. J Adv

Pharm Technol Res. 2012 Oct-Dec;3(4): 200–201. DOI: 10.4103/2231-4040.104709

- CK.Kamaraj. Certainty Vs. Clarity. Clearly Knowing 2021. Available online at: Certainty vs. Clarity (clearlyknowing.com)

- Hamish J Wilson. The myth of objectivity: is medicine moving towards a social constructivist medical paradigm? Family Practice 2000; 17: 203–209. DOI: 10.1093/fampra/17.2.203

- How heuristic thinking helps in reasoning logically. Harappa diaries 2020. Available online at: https://harappa.education/harappadiaries/meaning-of-a-heuristic-and-its-examples/

- Joachim P. Sturmberg, Carmel M. Martin. Complexity and health – yesterday's traditions, tomorrow's future. Journal of Evaluation in Clinical Practice. 2009; 15(3) 543–548. DOI: 10.1111/j.1365-2753.2009.01163.x

- Kim Krisberg. Narrative Medicine: Every Patient Has a Story. AAMC News 2017. Available online at: Narrative Medicine: Every Patient Has a Story | AAMC

- Padmanabhan V. Connecting with spiritual intelligence in medicine. Curr Med Issues 2021; 19:202-4. DOI: 10.4103/cmi.cmi_21_21

- Paul E Plsek, Trisha Greenhalgh. The challenge of complexity in health care. BMJ 2001; 323(7313): 625–628. DOI: 10.1136/bmj.323.7313.625 Available online at: https://www.researchgate.net/publication/232269387_Complexity_Science_The_Challenge_of_Complexity_in_Health_Care

- Sharma H. Meditation: Process and effects. Ayu 2015; 36:233-7 DOI: 10.4103/0974-8520.182756

#21: The need for psycho-spiritual history in clinical medicine

Introduction: In conventional modern medicine, while dealing with a new patient, it has been the practice to elicit details of the patient followed by details of the illness. The presenting symptoms in chronological order give an idea about the pathological process involved, which is further understood through a detailed history of present illness, the past history, the occupational, personal and family histories.

It is usual practice to proceed with understanding of the mental state in neurological and psychiatric illnesses. In diseases of the body where the pathogenesis is presumed to be a disorder of structure and/or function of one or more of its components, the psychological aspect of the patient is usually side-lined. More so, the spiritual aspect is out of consideration in conventional modern medicine.

There is a famous quote of Hippocrates [1]: 'It is more important to know what sort of person has a disease than to know what sort of disease a person has'. Here 'what sort of person' is about the psycho-spiritual aspect of the patient.

There are three components to patient care – the body component (structure-based), the mind-body component (thought-based) and the mind-body-spirit component (feeling-based). Conventional history taking is largely confined to the body component. Recently, understanding of the mind-body component has become mainstream [2], with emphasis on meditation, moderate exercise and stress management.

The role of the mind-body-spirit component in patient care is becoming increasingly recognized. The role of compassionate care of the patient in positively influencing the disease process from a distance (non-local) as well as from within the patient, has been observed [3]. Conversely, the presence of mind-body and the mind-body-spirit components in patient care indicate that human pathophysiology can result from absence of healthy mind and spirit in a patient.

In the presence of negative thoughts, the way a patient responds to a given treatment can be below expectations. Such negative thoughts can be recognized by probing into the patient's mental attitude. Similar is the adverse effect when the patient feels a lack of genuine love and understanding in one's social circle. Identifying these through a psycho-spiritual history helps to provide measures for restoring healthy mind and spirit in such patients, in addition to conventional treatment.

The average patient may not be forth-coming with the psycho-spiritual aspects of history, considering them to be too personal. Spending quality time with the patient with care and understanding, may encourage the patient to come out with these details. Two simple questions may help identify them – 1) Apart from the present disease, are you positive with other things in your life? 2) Do you feel adequately cared for by your relatives or friends?

Not recognising the presence of negativity in a patient's psycho-spiritual history can lead to inappropriate or ineffective treatment that may otherwise work well in a patient who has a positive attitude and has genuinely supportive people in one's life, a fact highlighted by the famous quote of Hippocrates.

Conclusion: While positivity and compassionate care of the patient are acknowledged to have a bearing on the disease outcome, conventional history-taking remains confined to aspects of body medicine. Inclusion of psycho-spiritual history in clinical medicine starting from the formative years of the medical student, leads to opening up of a hidden aspect of the patient's problem, which when tackled has significant therapeutic potential.

References:
[1] Hippocrates. Hippocrates - It is more important to know what sort of... (brainyquote.com)

[2] Brower V. Mind-body research moves towards the mainstream. EMBO Reports 2006; 7(4): 358–361. doi: 10.1038/sj.embor.7400671 https://www.ncbi.nlm.nih.gov/pmc/articles/PMC1456909/

[3] Vijayaraghavan P. A common platform for all systems of medicine. SCIREA Journal of Clinical Medicine 2023; 8(3), 176-180. doi: 10.54647/cm321071 SCIREA- Publisher of Open Access Journals

#22: Outline for Empathy-Based Medical Education

Introduction: Empathy, which is described as 'the ability to understand and share other people's feelings', has been recognized in recent years to play a central role for the successful practice of medicine. Hence, developing empathetic skills needs to be the underlying objective during the training of undergraduate medical students as well as in continuous education of health professionals.[1]

Drawbacks of present system: However, during the process of medical education, the quality of empathy that is naturally present within the student has been found to decline, since presently the process is 'left-brain dominated, analytical and evidence-based'.[2,3] While the goal of competence-based medical education is to ensure that 'all learners achieve the desired patient-centered outcomes during their training', all medical curricula including various versions of competence-based medical curriculum are taught based on a fixed schedule. This results in lot of stress for the students and is not conducive for fostering of empathy.

Bringing out latent empathy through self-directed learning: The task is to achieve the process of learning medicine and at the same time, preserve and foster the quality of empathy, present within the students. Towards this end, researchers have proposed a medical school curriculum that includes standardized patients and didactic sessions to teach empathy to medical students.[4] However, it is emphasized that there is a natural way to bring out the latent empathy from within students.

Spontaneous self-directed learning: Spontaneous learning based on one's own interest, is a form of self-directed learning that taps the student's sense of curiosity about the problem and concern for the patient. This natural method of learning is implemented right from the basic sciences, up to the final year clinical subjects. This entails the students to be exposed to actual cases in the OPD as well as the wards and allowing them to question and learn directly from the problems of the patient. For example, with respect to the subjects of Anatomy and Physiology, the patient diagnosed with a respiratory infection should prompt the study of the upper and lower respiratory tracts and their functional aspects. Students can observe and learn from teachers dealing with individual cases and in turn go about studying cases on their own with guidance from the teachers. Students learn about the structural and functional aspects in health and disease while remaining connected with the patients as individuals. Students learn about those topics that are applicable for individual cases and knowledge is acquired in a case-centered manner.

Purposeful acquisition of knowledge: Classroom

lectures can cover a broad outline of the subjects but having a fixed syllabus to be covered for each subject within a time frame is avoided. All evaluations to be done through case-based discussions, credits being given to the number of cases discussed in-depth with respect to each subject. The textbooks in each subject are to be treated as knowledge repositories for learning the topics relevant to the cases. The extent of theoretical knowledge the student acquires may be lesser than with a fixed syllabus, but whatever that is learnt in a patient-centered manner is more meaningful and stays longer. Knowledge acquired from textbooks will not be for reproducing them in the exams, thus avoiding the situation where the student is expected to absorb vast amounts of knowledge that remains unused.

Ensuring creativity and avoiding stress: While both textbooks and patients need to be studied side-by-side, studying primarily in a patient-centered manner as per one's own interest with the support of textbooks, helps to preserve and foster the quality of empathy. The 'self-directed spontaneous learning' ensures creativity in approach to problems, optimum utilization of one's time and avoids stress. The importance, intricacies and challenges of self-directed learning have been described,[5] but tapping the spiritual intelligence (relating to the 'inner self' or 'soul') of every student simplifies and facilitates self-directed learning from within.[6]

Cultivating the art of remaining focused: The student's connection with his or her own 'inner self' is crucial for a focused and creative mind; therefore, its cultivation through the process of meditation is particularly important. All medical schools can have spaces for meditation centres, where the techniques of meditation are taught and learnt. The emphasis will be on the art of remaining focused on the problems of the patient, while learning the theory behind them with teacher's guidance and the widely available digital resources.

Conclusion: The empathy-based medical education-EBME described above, facilitates the training of doctors who are competent as well as empathetic. It is finally a question of acquiring knowledge of the objective as well as the subjective aspect of medicine in a balanced manner. Keeping the subjective aspect as the base while acquiring the objective aspect, leads to balance between competence and empathy. The shift to an empathy-based curriculum, keeping in mind the immense benefits for the student as well as the patient, requires more of developing the attitude of being student and patient-centered rather than being disease-centered.

References:

1. Moudatsou M et al. The Role of Empathy in Health and Social Care Professionals. *Health Care (Basel).* 2020; 8(1):26 doi: 10.3390/healthcare8010026
https://www.ncbi.nlm.nih.gov/pmc/articles/PMC7151200/

2. Shelley, B. A value forgotten in doctoring: Empathy. *Arch Med Health Sci.* 2015; 3:169-73 doi: 10.4103/2321-4848.171895
https://journals.lww.com/armh/Fulltext/2015/03020/A_value_forgotten_in_doctoring__Empathy.1.aspx

3. Ahrweiler F et al. Determinants of physician empathy during medical education. *BMC Med Educ.* 2014; 14: 122. doi: 10.1186/1472-6920-14-122
https://www.ncbi.nlm.nih.gov/pmc/articles/PMC4080581/

4. Morris KE, Pappas TN. Creating a Medical School Curriculum to Teach Empathy. *Annals of Surgery Open.* 2021; 2(3): e085. doi: 10.1097/AS9.0000000000000085
https://www.ncbi.nlm.nih.gov/pmc/articles/PMC10455068/

5. Charokar K, Dulloo P. Self-directed Learning Theory to Practice. *J Adv Med Educ Prof.* 2022;

10(3): 135-144 doi: 10.30476/JAMP.2022.94833.1609
https://www.ncbi.nlm.nih.gov/pmc/articles/PMC9309162/

6. Padmanabhan V. Connecting with Spiritual Intelligence in Medicine. *Curr Med Issues.* 2021; 19(3):p 202-204 doi: 10.4103/cmi.cmi_21_21
https://journals.lww.com/cmii/Fulltext/2021/19030/Connecting_with_Spiritual_Intelligence_in_Medicine.17.aspx

#23: When 'Ignorance is Bliss' in Medicine

Introduction: Physicians hear occasional patients recalling with nostalgia that treatment of diseases was much simpler in good old days. Of late, the number of possibilities that need to be considered before coming to a diagnosis and start treatment have greatly increased for many diseases. However, in this age of spectacular medical advances, treatment of diseases can still be simple as well as effective with only limited medical knowledge; the statement 'ignorance is bliss' can indeed be true, provided the physician is connected with the 'pure consciousness' within himself (or herself), which is also the basis of everything in the universe.[1]

'Pure consciousness' as the source of healing: All newer methods of diagnosis and treatment are the outcome of 'scientific knowledge'. But 'knowledge' itself has its source from 'consciousness'. Of particular interest is that, the 'inner self' or 'pure consciousness' reached sub-consciously by every individual in the deep sleep state, has refreshing and healing qualities. This is within the experience of anyone who can find that the bliss felt after having a good sleep refreshes the mind, body and spirit. This healing 'inner self' is reached in the waking state, through the practice of meditation.[2]

'Being connected to the inner self' helps healing: The physician who is connected to the 'inner self', even if it is subconsciously, becomes part of the healing process. Many patients, if not all, are helped to move into a more blissful consciousness, through the positivity exhibited by such a physician. Invariably, every disease state is associated with consciousness that is restricted by the suffering caused by the disease process. For example, the patient suffering from neuropathic symptoms is constrained to be conscious of his burning feet and hence may lack the feeling of bliss. Apart from timely application of appropriate medical knowledge, the physician connected to his 'inner self' and enjoying the bliss therefrom, can help the patient to reach a more blissful state of consciousness through his verbal and body language. This would facilitate healing of all types of diseases and with proper guidance, even encourage the patient to connect with his own healing 'inner self'. While some physicians may find connecting with 'inner self' to be easy and simple through a good sleep or through meditation, many will find that learning meditation is only another skill that needs to be mastered.

'Simple' or 'scientific' knowledge, makes no difference: While mind-body therapies [3] are patient-dependent self-help strategies, the physician who is connected with his own 'inner self' directly helps to initiate the healing process. Positivity is manifested by the physician regardless of whether the medical knowledge utilized is 'simple' or the more complex 'scientific' knowledge, which gives greater understanding of the disease and its treatment. Another way of looking at it is that the blissful physician who is connected to his 'inner self' can easily empathize with the patient, thus helping the patient to develop faith in the treating physician, which in-turn leads to healing through in-born mechanisms.[4]

Conclusion: In medicine, 'ignorance is bliss' when the source of healing, the 'pure consciousness' or 'inner self', is connected with by the physician and made use of. There may be 'ignorance' of complex 'scientific knowledge', but there is 'wisdom' of being connected with the source of all healing, which makes application of even 'simple knowledge' often effective. Constantly reaching out for the state of 'pure consciousness' through practice of meditation, allows him to remain connected with the source of healing. Regular practice of meditation can thus be a meaningful part of learning and become a valuable adjunct for the practice of medicine.

References:

1. Deepak Chopra. The Seven Spiritual Laws of Success. The Washington Post 1994. WashingtonPost.com: The Seven Spiritual

Laws of Success: A Practical Guide to the Fulfillment of Your Dreams
https://www.washingtonpost.com/wp-srv/style/longterm/books/chap1/sevenspirituallaws.htm#TOP

2. Sharma H. Meditation: Process and effects Ayu. 2015; 36:233–7 doi: 10.4103/0974-8520.182756
https://www.ncbi.nlm.nih.gov/pmc/articles/PMC4895748/

3. Mary Koithan. The Inner Healer; Mind-Body Strategies for Health. J Nurse Pract. 2009; 5(5): 374–375. doi:10.1016/j.nurpra.2009.01.012
https://www.ncbi.nlm.nih.gov/pmc/articles/PMC2754856/

4. Albert wang. Psychoneuroimmunology: A New Approach to Curing Diseases 2016. https://sites.bu.edu/ombs/2016/02/05/psychoneuroimmunology-a-new-approach-to-curing-diseases

#24: Science that swears by objectivity is half-blind

Introduction: Objective and subjective are terms used to either accept or reject ideas in scientific literature. But on scrutiny, such usage seems to be based on certain questionable assumptions.

No objectivity without an element of subjectivity: It is widely understood that science is knowledge that is based on a systematic and objective study of the natural world. However, such a study is conducted by the human being, who is a combination of objectivity and subjectivity. Whatever is deemed to be objective, is in the final analysis, the subjective opinion of an individual. Thus, there can be no objectivity without an element of subjectivity.

The role of common sense: Thus science, by its very origin, has a subjective element. Though its boundaries are not clearly defined, science has proved to be immensely useful to mankind and has been the basis of great technological progress. This has been possible because the human being is endowed with a third quality, which is common sense. Common sense allows a balanced approach, where objectivity and subjectivity are treated equally without any bias. Without common sense, scientists can lose touch with reality and end up building castles in the air. Objectivity is the engine of science but subjectivity is the rail on which it runs.

Thus objectivity, subjectivity and common sense need to be viewed as means for grasping the truth, with each by itself throwing some light on the hitherto unrevealed truth. The three together form the basis of an unseen natural methodology that helps to reveal truth.

Too much of objectivity can stall meaningful progress: The tendency to become too objective is the bane of science. It can stall meaningful progress and makes the scientist and science to go around in circles. Usually, any new discovery in science is considered 'scientific' only if it can be shown to be true in the form of some mathematical equation. But the subtle point here is that even mathematical equations that appear objective, have a subjective element.

The classic example is the case of quantum mechanics (which is about indeterminism in physical laws). It is well known among physicists that the equations of quantum mechanics 'work', but all agree that it is not known 'how they work'. There is general conclusion that it is not necessary to understand 'how they work', but nevertheless it makes sense to use the equations since they actually 'work' in the real world [1].

Objective evidence and subjective experience: There is another aspect of science that is less well known. It has become an established norm that any scientific conclusion needs to be supported by 'objective' evidence. Something is accepted as objective if several people subjectively agree that it is 'objective'. However, a rational conclusion perceived internally within one's subjective 'experience' and supported by several people who agree with a similar 'experience', is dismissed as being 'merely subjective'.

Focusing within the three sides of objectivity, subjectivity and common sense: It is clear that overemphasis on subjectivity can lead to dilution of objectivity in scientific studies. However, scientific studies still make sense when the focus is within the boundaries formed by objectivity, subjectivity and common sense. Such an approach can be the basis of a practical methodology that allows intuition and creativity to express themselves. Equanimity will ensure this focus, with no place given for excessive tilt towards any one side.

Conclusion: There are enough reasons to consider objectivity and subjectivity on an even scale [2]. Scientists who swear by objectivity and reject subjectivity do a great disservice to the progress of the 'search for truth in the natural world' if that is what science is about. Albert Einstein has famously said that 'imagination is more important than knowledge' [3]. Great scientific discoveries have been made based on intuition (which is subjective), that has been further pursued with objectivity and common sense. To swear by objectivity can be a personal choice but science cannot remain half-blind for that reason.

References:

[1] The Trouble with Quantum Mechanics. Steven Weinberg, 2017. http://quantum.phys.unm.edu/466-17/QuantumMechanicsWeinberg.pdf

[2] Smith, H. F. (1999). Subjectivity and Objectivity in Analytic Listening. Journal of the American Psychoanalytic Association, 47(2), 465-484. doi: 10.1177/00030651990470022101
https://pubmed.ncbi.nlm.nih.gov/10422050/

[3] Imagination is more important than knowledge. Nucleus_AI, 2023. https://yourstory.com/2023/05/transformative-power-imagination

#25: The 'Inside-Out' Approach to Therapeutic Care

1. Introduction:

Practice of modern medicine has transitioned from being mainly body medicine, to inclusion of mind-body medicine, to the recent recognition of mind-body-spirit medicine. Medicine is taught to students and is convenient to practice, when health and disease processes are considered as consequences of function or dysfunction of body parts. The more advanced concept of mind-body medicine is put to use when the influence of thoughts on the body's functioning is harnessed [1]. The practice of medicine becomes even more subtle, when the reality of mind-body-spirit medicine cognized by the physician, helps him to address the emotional and spiritual aspects of the disease process [2].

2. The 'outside-in' approach:

Even though these three layers of cognition exist, in actual practice, the first or body medicine carries most weightage for the patient as well as the physician. The patient is first interested in getting relief from the problem afflicting one's body, before dealing with the mind-body or mind-body-spirit aspects of the problem, and would expect the physician to do the same. From the diagnostic viewpoint, this 'outside-in' approach helps the physician to quickly connect with the patient, while the disease process is being understood.

3. Focusing on the patients thought and feeling:

While causation of disease at the physical level is known to be due to various factors, it is increasingly known that the source of many diseases lies in failure of the individual to cope with the stress of day-to-day life at the mental and spiritual level. Either the patient lacks positivity of mind or feels a lack of inner joy, often one leading to the other. The problem in the 'mindset' or 'inner being', that results in the patient falling ill, is understood by taking a psycho-spiritual history [3].

4. 'Dis-ease' of 'inner being':

Non communicable diseases like hypertension and diabetes have been shown to occur due to the patient adopting an adverse life style that reflects a problem in the 'inner being' [4]. Infections are known to set in when the patient is stressed [5]. Likewise, there is plenty of evidence in recent times for the role of the mind in disease processes [6]. A caring environment that supports positive thought and preserves inner joy, thus keeps most of the diseases at bay.

5. The 'inside-out' approach:

Therefore, for many illnesses it makes therapeutic sense when the problem occurring in the thought and feeling of the patient is first understood and set right. This 'inner being' focused approach, tackles the root of the disease [7], making rest of the therapy related to the body, simpler and more effective. Understanding the 'inner being' of the patient would thus be a valuable clinical skill for the physician, while dealing with any type of case.

6. Conclusion:

While most patients expect immediate relief related to the body, adopting the 'inside-out' approach to therapeutic care makes sense once there is promise of wholesome healing of body, mind and spirit. Health care systems can thus become more meaningful, with minimal use of diagnostic or therapeutic intervention. The following quote of Dr. Bernard Lown sums up the matter: 'Do as much as possible *for* the patient and as little as possible *to* the patient'.

References:

[1] John A. Astin, Shauna L. Shapiro, David M. Eisenberg, Kelly L. Forys. Mind-Body Medicine: State of the Science, Implications for Practice. *The Journal of the American Board of Family Practice* Mar

2003, 16 (2) 131-147; DOI: 10.3122/jabfm.16.2.131 Mind-Body Medicine: State of the Science, Implications for Practice | American Board of Family Medicine

[2] Glenis Mark, Antonia Lyons. Conceptualizing Mind, Body, Spirit Interconnections Through, and Beyond, Spiritual Healing Practices. 2014, *Explore* 10 (5), 294-299; DOI: 10.1016/j.explore.2014.06.003. https://www.sciencedirect.com/science/article/pii/S1550830714001098

[3] Padmanabhan, V. The Need for Psycho-Spiritual History in Clinical Medicine. *Clinical Medicine And Health Research Journal.* 2023, *3*(5), 522–523. DOI: 10.18535/cmhrj.v3i5.222 https://cmhrj.com/index.php/cmhrj/article/view/222

[4] Glass DR. Lifestyle medicine: A positive approach to stemming the tide of non-communicable diseases in South Africa. *S Afr Fam Pract (2004)* 2021, 26;63(1):e1-e4. DOI: 10.4102/safp.v63i1.5394. PMID: 34797100; PMCID: PMC8603158. Lifestyle medicine: A positive approach to stemming the tide of non-communicable diseases in South Africa - PMC

[5] Cohen S. Psychosocial Influences on Immunity and Infectious Disease in Humans. *Handbook of*

Human Stress and Immunity. 1994:301–19. DOI: 10.1016/B978-0-12-285960-1.50016-2. Epub 2014 Jun 27. PMCID: PMC7150128. Psychosocial Influences on Immunity and Infectious Disease in Humans - PMC

[6] Brower V. Mind-body research moves towards the mainstream. *Embo Rep.* 2006 Apr;7(4):358-61. DOI:10.1038/sj.embor.7400671. PMID: 16585935; PMCID: PMC1456909. https://pmc.ncbi.nlm.nih.gov/articles/PMC1456909/

[7] Prabakar AD. The Power of Thought: The Role of Psychological Attentiveness and Emotional Support in Patient Trajectories. *Yale J Biol Med.* 2024 Sep 30;97(3):335-347. DOI: 10.59249/CPTG1770. PMID: 39351320; PMCID: PMC11426302. https://pmc.ncbi.nlm.nih.gov/articles/PMC11426302/

Bibliography

1: Health Care Needs a Fundamentally New Approach - Published in Futurehealth.org, Sept. 2010

2: The Unlimited Potential of Mind-Body-Spirit Medicine - Published in Futurehealth.org, May 2010

3: Everything is a Play of Consciousness - Published in Futurehealth.org, June 2010

4: Our Built-in Biofeedback - Published in Futurehealth.org, May 2010

5: Understanding Meditation - Published in Futurehealth.org, July 2010

6: Bliss Feedback Therapy - Published in Futurehealth.org, August 2010

7: When Consciousness Becomes the Basis of Structure - Published in Futurehealth.org, Sept. 2011

8: Three Intelligences and Three Tendencies - Published in Futurehealth.org, Feb. 2012

9: Improving the Quality of Health Care from Within - Published in Futurehealth.org, April 2012

10: Becoming Aware of Mind-Body-Spirit Medicine - Published in Futurehealth.org, April 2014

11: Empathy, Research and the Medical Teacher - Published in Docplexus.in, Sept. 2015

12: Fixing the Basic flaw in Medical Education and Health Care - Published in Opednews.com, July 2016

13: Intuitive Medicine - Published in International Journal of Medical Research Professionals, March 2017

14: Quantum View of Medicine and its Implications - Published in International Journal of Academic Medicine, Jan 2018

15: The Need for Empathy-Based Medical Education – Published in Archives of Medicine & Health Sciences,

June 2019

16: Halting Dehumanization in Medicine – Published in International Journal of Academic Medicine, Mar 2020

17: Connecting with Spiritual Intelligence in Medicine – Published in Current Medical Issues, July 2021

18: Consciousness as the basis of disease and disaster – Published in European Journal of Biomedical and Pharmaceutical Sciences, July 2022

#19: A common platform for all systems of medicine – Published in SCIREA Journal of Clinical Medicine, May 2023

#20: Clarity as against Certainty in Medicine – Published in International Journal of Development Research, May 2023

#21: The need for psycho-spiritual history in clinical medicine – Published in Clinical Medicine and Health Research Journal, Sept. 2023

#22: Outline for Empathy-Based Medical Education – Published in Clinical Medicine and Health Research Journal, Jan 2024

#23: When 'Ignorance is Bliss' in Medicine – Published in International Journal of Science and Research, June 2025

#24: Science that swears by objectivity is half-blind – Published in International Journal of Innovative Research in Medical Science, Nov 2024

#25: The 'Inside-Out' Approach to Therapeutic Care – Published in International Journal of Science and Research, April 2025

ABOUT THE AUTHOR

Dr Vijayaraghavan Padmanabhan MD lives in Chennai, India. He graduated from Madras Medical College, where even as a student he was interested in the philosophical aspects of Medicine. His interactions with Sri Sathya Sai Baba strengthened his spiritual moorings and inspired him to write the first article, which was blessed by Him. He is a former Professor of Medicine at Madras Medical College, Chennai and Associate Professor of Medicine at ESIC Medical College & Hospital, Chennai, India.

AFTERWORD

This book has been an attempt to bring out the finer aspects of medicine, often considered subjective and lying unseen within the mind-occupying grosser aspects. If the book reveals a fresh perspective to medicine for the reader, it would have served its purpose. The Author requests the reader to share the good word, and leave a review on the Amazon store page of this book.

BOOKS BY THIS AUTHOR

Spirituality For The Modern Mind:

Why isn't believing in God a superstition? Why doesn't God intervene more often to make things perfect? What makes humans need to worship something outside of themselves? Is morality a restrictive thing? How is ethics beneficial to humans? Will AI ever become a threat to humanity; why or why not? What will make me proud to be human in a world increasingly driven by AI in the next 5 years? Could global empathy ever be taught? What is the main thing to do for peace in the world? How can we find and use the real power of the mind? Is spirituality inherent to the human condition, or does it require specific practice? If the world is inherently suffering, why did God put me here in the first place? This book deals with these and several such questions that explore human nature and existence, and suggests ways to come out of the multiple crises of our times…

Partyless Governance - A Vision for a Better World:

The present day world is ridden with crises. We have pieces instead of Peace. There is perpetual tussle going on between different forces at the global level. While there is spiritual awakening and a transformation in the collective consciousness, we need a vision for an alternative system of governance that is truly integrative and promotes the values of Truth, Love and Peace. This book addresses this need by suggesting Partyless Governance that is conscience-based, as an alternative to the present party-based governance that is ideology-based.

Musings on Ideal Democracy - Q&A on Partyless Governance:

What power does a voting citizen have today? What can citizens do to vitalize our democracy? Can politics be spiritualized? Can Advaita Vedanta be a stronger foundation for Democracy as mentioned by Dr. Ambedkar? Is it possible to eliminate political parties in the democratic system? Does capitalism pose an existential threat to humanity? Are all levels of inequality consistent with a healthy, well-functioning democracy? Is identity politics regressive in nature? Which concept ought to be given more priority, development or democracy? Can democracy and development go together? Is there a link between 'climate change' and democracy? This book deals with several such questions concerning governance and suggests that matters concerning Democracy stand simplified from the point of view of oneness of the soul, achievable through Partyless Governance, that is conscience-based.

www.ingramcontent.com/pod-product-compliance
Lightning Source LLC
Chambersburg PA
CBHW071414210526
45465CB00001B/389